PATHOGENESIS AND TREATMENT OF DIABETES MELLITUS

Pathogenesis and Treatment of Diabetes Mellitus

edited by

J.K. RADDER
H.H.P.J. LEMKES
H.M.J. KRANS

Department of Endocrinology and Metabolism
Leiden University Hospital
Leiden, The Netherlands

1986 **MARTINUS NIJHOFF PUBLISHERS**
a member of the KLUWER ACADEMIC PUBLISHERS GROUP
BOSTON / DORDRECHT / LANCASTER

Distributors

for the United States and Canada: Kluwer Academic Publishers, 101 Philip Drive, Assinippi Park, Norwell, MA 02061, USA
for the UK and Ireland: Kluwer Academic Publishers, MTP Press Limited, Falcon House, Queen Square, Lancaster LA1 1RN, UK
for all other countries: Kluwer Academic Publishers Group, Distribution Center, P.O. Box 322, 3300 AH Dordrecht, The Netherlands

Library of Congress Cataloging in Publication Data

Pathogenesis and treatment of diabetes mellitus.

    Based on a Boerhaave course organized by the Faculty of Medicine, University of Leiden, the Netherlands.
    Includes index.
    I. Radder, Jasper Katrinus. II. Lemkes, H.H.P.J.
III. Krans, Hendrik Michiel Jan. IV. Rijksuniversiteit te Leiden. Faculteit der Geneeskunde. [DNLM:
1. Diabetes Mellitus--etiology--congresses. 2. Diabetes Mellitus--therapy--congresses. WK 810 P2974]
RC660.A15P38 1986   616.4'62   86-18129

ISBN-13: 978-94-010-8411-6   e-ISBN-13: 978-94-009-4301-8
DOI: 10.1007978-94-009-4301-8

Copyright

Foreword

In this book on diabetes mellitus both the pathogenesis and treatment of the disease will be discussed.
Pathogenetic studies have led to the distinction between type I and type II diabetes. In type I hyperglycaemia is due predominantly to insulin deficiency; in type II insulin resistance is more important.

Three pathogenetic factors are thought to play a role in the etiology of type I diabetes: heredity, viral infections and immunity. There may be a relationship between these three aspects since genetic predisposition changes the susceptibility to viral infections and/or the immunological defence against these infections. Insulitis ensues. Autoimmune processes initiated by this chain of events may contribute to the destruction of the B cells in the islets of Langerhans and diabetes may eventually follow. This means that at the time of the sudden outbreak of the disease, the destructive process has already been active for years.

With respect to clinical medicine several questions arise. Does the above mentioned chain of events inevitably lead to clinically manifest diabetes mellitus? Is it possible to detect such a development at an early stage? And if so, is it worthwhile as far as preventive or therapeutic measures, such as vaccination or immunosuppressive therapy, are concerned? Are such measures still useful when the disease is full blown? Is genetic counseling possible and warranted in view of our present knowledge and which markers could be used?

After a short introduction of Dr. J.K. Radder, Drs. J.E. Craighead, G.F. Bottazzo and R.B. Tattersall and their coworkers will discuss several aspects of the pathogenesis of type I diabetes and the possible clinical consequences.

Insulin resistance is a well-recognized feature of type II diabetes. The resistance can be localized at three distinct levels: in B cells in the islets of Langerhans, in the target tissues of insulin and, thirdly, at an intermediary level, notably as anti-insulin antibodies in the blood, as antibodies against the insulin receptor and as elevated levels of the counterregulatory hormones.

During the last decade it has become clear that the regulation of metabolism is in fact a fine tuning of the complementary actions of the neural and hormonal systems. In the central nervous system the hypothalamus is regarded as an important integrating station. However, while our understanding of peripheral activation by the autonomic nervous system is fairly advanced, the involvement of the central mechanism in the activation of the islets of Langerhans is not yet clear and therefore the influence of the central nervous system on insulin resistance is still questioned.

Dr. H.M.J. Krans will introduce this subject, which will be discussed then in more detail by Drs. M.A. Pfeifer, P.J. Lefebvre, A.B. Steffens and Tj. Wieringa and their coworkers.

The treatment of diabetes mellitus with diet, or oral hypoglycaemic agents and insulin has changed considerably in the past few years. These changes can be attributed both to the above mentioned new insights into the pathogenesis of the disease and to the endeavour to achieve normoglycaemia in order to prevent or retard neurovascular complications. Another topic will be the intentionally more fysiological approach: the pancreas transplantation.

Dietary advice is still one of the pillars of the treatment of diabetes mellitus, in addition to the prescription of hypoglycaemic agents and education of the patient in order to provide insight into the influence of stress and exercise on the metabolic control of diabetes. The approach of dieting is different for the two types of diabetes: in type I it is adjustment of the distribution of the meals and in type II it is adaptation of the quantity of energy to needs.

Our insight into the influence of various carbohydrates on the blood glucose level has changed drastically in the last years: sugar (saccharose) is no longer forbidden and carbohydrates in leguminous plants are preferred. Which mechanisms determine the effects of the carbohydrates in various foodstuffs? Has diet, and notably the use of polyunsaturated fatty acids, a specific purpose in the treatment of (the vascular complications of) diabetes?

Oral hypoglycaemic agents, sulfonylurea derivatives as well as biguanides, lower the blood glucose level. In addition to the B cell stimulating effect of the first group of agents, both exert an extrapancreatic influence, notably their "insulin-like" effect on the cells of the target tissues of insulin. An important question for the practitioner is whether the advantages of lowering blood glucose level counterbalance the reported disadvantages of inducing cardiovascular disease.

These subjects are introduced by Dr. J.L. Touber and discussed in more detail by Drs. D.J.A. Jenkins and H. Keen and their coworkers.

Conventional treatment of diabetes with insulin makes use of the subcutaneous route. The maintenance of normoglycaemia under these conditions often leads to peripheral hyperinsulinaemia. The effects of long-term hyperinsulinaemia, however, are poorly understood. Moreover subcutaneous insulin delivery does not result in a normal portal-peripheral insulin gradient. It may also be questioned whether control of glucose metabolism by means of exogenous insulin can ever be physiological since it is based on signals derived from the concentration of glucose in the peripheral blood. Not only the cephalic phase reflex responses to sensory stimuli (the sight and smell of food) but probably also the interactions between the central and peripheral nervous systems and gastrointestinal hormones may determine the appropriate timing for and quantity of insulin to be delivered from the B cells. Therefore an adequately programmed administration of insulin might offer an effective means of controlling blood glucose levels. Qualitatively the normal portal-peripheral insulin gradient and the normal physiological pattern of insulin secretion must be included in this programme.

This section will focus on the possible consequences of hyper-insulinaemia and alternative means of insulin delivery. It is introduced by Dr. J. Terpstra and discussed in more detail by Drs. E.R. Trimble, D.R. Matthews, A.M. Albisser and coworkers.

Transplantation of the pancreas is emerging from the experimental stage. In centres with experience the 1-2 years survival rate of the transplant has increased from 25 to 40%. For the time being this procedure is still reserved for patients on immunosuppressive therapy because of concomitant renal transplantation.

As far as the physiological functioning of the transplant is concerned it should be kept in mind that the denervated tail of the pancreas, now stripped of its exocrine function, is connected directly with the peripheral circulation.

Dr. H.H.P.J. Lemkes will introduce this subject which is reviewed by Dr. P. McMaster.

Contents

Foreword   V

Part   1.   : Pathogenesis of Diabetes Mellitus

Section   1.1. : Type I Diabetes Mellitus
Chapter   1.1.1.: Introduction: Type I Diabetes Mellitus
                   J.K. Radder   1
           1.1.2.: Autoimmune pathogenesis of viral diabetes
                   P.G. Babu, S.A. Huber and J.E. Graighead   11
           1.1.3.: Immunological features of insulin-dependent diabetes
                   mellitus
                   F. Becker and G.F. Bottazzo   16
           1.1.4.: Genetic counselling in Diabetes Mellitus
                   R.B. Tattersall   27

Section   1.2. : Type II Diabetes Mellitus
Chapter   1.2.1.: Introduction: Pathogenesis of type II Diabetes
                   Mellitus
                   H.M.J. Krans   33
           1.2.2.: Insulin secretion in noninsulin-dependent Diabetes
                   Mellitus
                   V. Broadstone, W.K. Ward, J.C. Beard, J.D. Best,
                   J.B. Halter, R. Judzewitsch, D. Porte and M.A.
                   Pfeifer   39
           1.2.3.: Insulin antagonism
                   P.J. Lefebvre and A.S. Luyckx   58
           1.2.4.: The contribution of the central nervous system to
                   the regulation of insulin release and the stabiliza-
                   tion of blood glucose
                   A.B. Steffens and P.G.M. Luiten   63
           1.2.5.: Cellular insulin resistance
                   Tj. Wieringa   75

Part   2.   : Treatment of Diabetes Mellitus

Section   2.1. : Diet and hypoglycaemic agents
Chapter   2.1.1.: Introduction: Diet and hypoglycaemic agents
                   J.L. Touber   83
           2.1.2.: Diet and Diabetes
                   R.G. Josse, A.L. Jenkins and D.J.A. Jenkins   91
           2.1.3.: Oral hypoglycaemic drugs
                   H. Keen and S. Ng Tang Fui   103

X

Section   2.2.   : Insulin
Chapter   2.2.1.: Introduction: Insulin treatment
                    J. Terpstra   121
            2.2.2.: Hyperinsulinaemia
                    E.R. Trimble   123
            2.2.3.: Insulin: The physiological basis of its administration
                    D.R. Matthews   131
            2.2.4.: Diabetes Technology: From the pump to the micro-
                    processor
                    A.M. Albisser and B.S. Leibel   142

Section   2.3.   : Pancreas transplantation
Chapter   2.3.1.: Introduction: Pancreas transplantation
                    H.H.P.J. Lemkes   152
            2.3.2.: Current state of pancreas transplantation
                    P. McMaster, W.A. Jurewics, B.H. Gunson, R.M.
                    Kirby   156

Index of subjects   167

List of the addresses of the contributors
(and their co-workers)

A.M. Albisser (and B.S. Leibel).
Div. of Biomedical Research, Hospital for Sick Children, 555 University Avenue, Toronto, Ontario M5G 1X8, Canada.

G.F. Bottazzo (and F. Becker).
Dept. of Immunology, Arthur Stanley House, The Middlesex Hospital Medical School, 40-50 Tottenham Street, London W1P 9PG, United Kingdom.

J.E. Graighead (and P.G. Babu and S.A. Huber).
Dept. of Pathology, University of Vermont, College of Medicine, Burlington VT 05405, U.S.A.

D.J.A. Jenkins (and R.G. Josse and A.L. Jenkins).
Dept. of Nutritional Science, Faculty of Medicine, Fitzgerald Building, 150 College Street, Toronto, Ontario M5S 1A8, Canada.

H. Keen (and S. Ng Tang Fui).
Dept. of Medicine, Unit for Metab. Med., 4th floor, Hunts House, Guy's Hospital, London Bridge SE1 9RT, United Kingdom.

H.M.J. Krans.
Dept. of Endocrinology and Metabolism, University Hospital, P.O. box 9600, 2300 RC Leiden, The Netherlands.

H.H.P.J. Lemkes.
Dept. of Endocrinology and Metabolism, University Hospital, P.O. box 9600, 2300 RC Leiden, The Netherlands.

P.J. Lefebvre (and A.S. Luyckx*).
Institut de Medicine, Hôpital de Bavière, 66 Boulevard de la Constitution, B-4000 Luik, Belgium.

D.R. Matthews.
Diabetes Research Lab., University of Oxford, Nuffield Department of Clinical Medicine. Radcliffe Infirmary, Woodstock Road, Oxford OX2 6HE, United Kingdom.

P. McMaster (and W.A. Jurewics, B.H. Gunson and R.M. Kirby).
Queen Elisabeth Hospital, Edgbaston, Birmingham B15 2TH, United Kingdom.

---

* deceased in 1985

M.A. Pfeifer (and V. Broadstone, W.K. Ward, J.C. Beard, J.D. Best, J.B. Halter, R. Judzewitsch and D. Porte).
VA Medical Centre, Medical Services, 800 Zorn Avenue, Louisville KY 40202, U.S.A.

J.K. Radder.
Dept. of Endocrinology and Metabolism, University Hospital, P.O. Box 9600, 2300 RC Leiden, The Netherlands.

A.B. Steffens (and P.G.M. Luiten).
Zoological Lab., Kerklaan 30, 9751 NN Haren (Gr), The Netherlands.

R.B. Tattersall.
Dept. of Medicine Ward C54, University Hospital, Queen's Medical Centre, Nottingham, NG7 2UH, United Kingdom.

J. Terpstra.
Dept. of Endocrinology and Metabolism, University Hospital, P.O. Box 9600, 2300 RC Leiden, The Netherlands.

J.L. Touber.
Dept. of Int. Medicine, University Hospital (AMC), Meibergdreef 9, 1105 AZ Amsterdam, The Netherlands.

Tj. Wieringa.
Dept. of Endocrinology and Metabolism, University Hospital, P.O. Box 9600, 2300 RC Leiden, The Netherlands.

1. Pathogenesis of Diabetes Mellitus

1.1. Type I Diabetes Mellitus

1.1.1. Introduction: Type I Diabetes Mellitus

J.K. Radder

1. INTRODUCTION

Diabetes mellitus is defined by the WHO (1) as a state of chronic hyperglycaemia. The main hypoglycaemic factor, insulin, is a hormone produced by the B-cells of the islets of Langerhans in the pancreas. An increase in the blood glucose level leads to insulin secretion. Insulin exerts its hypoglycaemic effect by suppressing glucose production in the liver and by stimulating glucose uptake in fat and muscle after binding to a specific receptor in the cell membrane. By means of this feedback loop glucose homeostasis is ensured. Hyperglycaemia can thus be caused by a decreased insulin production or a diminished insulin action or both. Other hormonal and neural influences can modulate this system.

From the clinical point of view diabetes mellitus can be distinguished in the lean, ketosis-prone, juvenile-onset and the obese, non-ketosis-prone, maturity-onset form, now called type I and type II diabetes, respectively (see table I). This distinction between the two types appeared also to have pathogenetic significance. In type I diabetes hyperglycaemia is due predominantly to insulin deficiency; in type II insulin resistance is more important. Therefore, as far as the treatment is concerned, type I diabetes is insulin-dependent and type II is non-insulin-dependent.

Apart from these two forms of idiopathic diabetes mellitus hyperglycaemia can be malnutrition-related or associated with certain conditions and syndromes, such as pancreatic disease, diseases of hormonal etiology, drug- or chemical-induced conditions, abnormalities of insulin or its receptor and certain genetic syndromes (2). The recognition of the several forms of diabetes mellitus has led to the notion that diabetes mellitus is not a disease with a single etiology, i.e. it is not a pathogenetic entity, but that it is a heterogeneous disorder with several causes leading to hyperglycaemia, i.e. it is a syndrome, like for instance anaemia. This increase in our knowledge has given rise to many fruitful investigations and new insights into the etiology and pathogenesis of diabetes mellitus.

TABLE

CHARACTERISTICS OF TYPE I (INSULIN-DEPENDENT)
AND TYPE II (NON-INSULIN-DEPENDENT) DIABETES

CHARACTERISTIC	TYPE I	TYPE II
Weight at onset	non-obese	often obese
Age at onset	usually < 30 years	usually > 40 years
Peak age	12-14 years	65 years
Incidence	$11/10^5$ (< 20 years)	?
Seasonal variation	present	? absent
Prevalence	0,5%	2%
Sex	slight male predominance	female predominance
Onset	rapid-gradual symptoms severe	mild; insidious incidental finding
Ketosis	usual	uncommon
Remission	often occurs	? absent
Duration at onset of late complications	usually several years	may be present at diagnosis

2. CLINIC OF TYPE I DIABETES

Type I diabetes mellitus usually develops before the age of 20 with a peak around puberty. The complaints are polydipsia, polyuria, hyperphagia, weight loss, visual disturbances and genital infections. It can also occur, however, at older ages. The younger the patient the shorter the period of symptoms. Insulin therapy should be started in these cases as soon as possible in order to prevent severe ketoacidosis, coma and eventually death. For some of the older patients initially a diet alone or a diet in combination with a sulfonylurea drug may be sufficient. However, by definition all patients should be insulin-dependent within a year.

A slight male preponderance is found in type I diabetes. In mice it has been reported that the male sex hormone may help to induce diabetes mellitus (3). However, when accompanied by other autoimmune endocrine disorders, such as Hashimoto's or Addison's diseases, type I diabetes is more likely to develop in women. Becker and colleagues (see chapter 1.1.3.) propose on account of this and other characteristics that two types of type I diabetes: type I a and type I b can be distinguished. They call type I a "juvenile-onset" and type I b "polyendocrine".

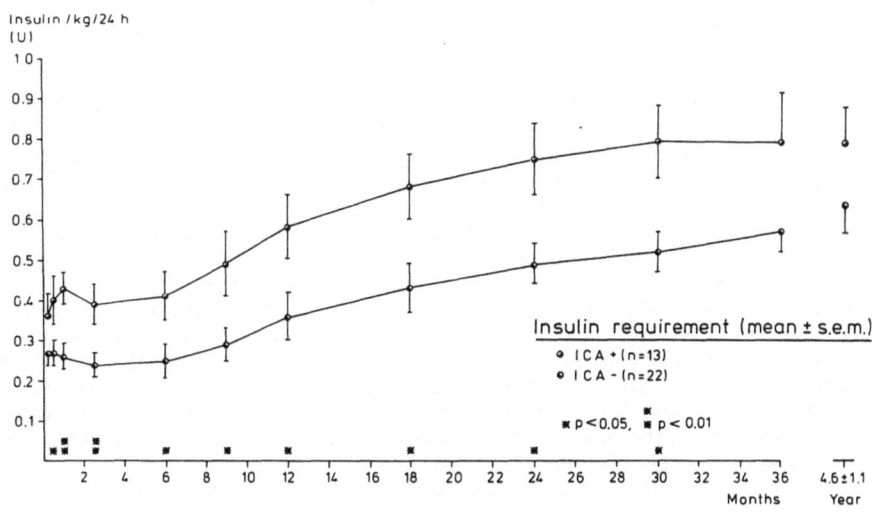

FIGURE 1. Insulin requirement (U/kg/24 h) in islet cell antibody positive (ICA+) (n = 13) and negative (ICA-) (n = 22) type I diabetics in the first 36 months and 4.6 ± 1.1 years after diagnosis.

In spite of the abrupt onset of the symptoms of the disease a long asymptomatic period before the clinical outbreak of the disease has been reported. Srikanta et al. (4, 5) showed in 4 twins, of whom 3 were islet cell antibody (ICA) positive for more than 5 years, a progressive decline in first phase insulin response to intravenous glucose before they developed typical type I diabetes. A slight increase in the fasting blood glucose and glucose intolerance were only seen shortly before the outbreak of clinical type I diabetes. In families with a type I diabetic complement fixing ICA (CF-ICA) have been detected in non-diabetic siblings, who share one or both HLA-haplotypes with their diabetic brother or sister (6). It has been found that about 50% of these non-diabetic sibs will develop type I diabetes (7, 8). (CF-)ICA and HLA may thus predict the outbreak of the disease.

A seasonal variation in the incidence of type I diabetes with a peak in the winter, has been observed in children of more than 5 years old (9) - suggesting a viral etiology of the disease. However, a direct relation between the clinical onset of type I diabetes and a viral infection could be confirmed only in a few cases (10, 11). In most cases an infectious disease merely seems to provoke the clinical manifestation of type I diabetes. This agrees with the concept of a long asymptomatic period, which means that the initial etiological damage to the B-cells of the islets of Langerhans must have occurred years ago.

The course of the disease varies markedly among the patients. A "honeymoon period" (i.e. a partial remission) usually occurs. But the length of the period differs from patient to patient. A complete remission is rare. The degree and duration of the remission are related to the endogenous insulin reserve. In a group of 40 type I diabetics, 11 females and 29 males, with a mean age of 27 years we found that in the ICA positive group (37% of total) the insulin requirement in the first five years after diagnosis was higher (fig. 1) and that 4.5 years after diagnosis the C-peptide reaction after glucagon stimulation was lower (fig. 2) than in the ICA negative group. The patients who developed insulin antibodies (34% of total) had also a higher insulin requirement (fig. 3) and a lower C-peptide reaction (fig. 4). The metabolic control did not differ significantly between the groups.

After the remission period, when the patient produces no longer (endogenous) insulin, the required insulin dose is still different. If the insulin requirement is higher than· was expected on the basis of the endogenous insulin reserve, then insulin resistance may exist. In this respect circulating insulin antagonists, like insulin antibodies, insulin receptor antibodies or growth hormone, or other factors, may be incriminated (see chapter 1.2.3.).

Most patients with type I diabetes acquire the neurovascular complications of the disease, but the manifestation and severity of these complications differ from one patient to the next. In addition to the influence of the metabolic control on the development of these complications, constitutional factors seem to play a role. Specific HLA antigens have been found to be associated with more severe complications (12).

With respect to genetic counselling most questions are asked by future parents with type I diabetes. They are concerned about the chance that their children will acquire the disease at a young age. Because the genetic transmission of type I diabetes is basically unknown the genetic advice emanates from empirical data.

3. PATHOGENESIS OF TYPE I DIABETES

The insulin deficiency of type I diabetes is caused by B-cell destruction. Three etiological factors may play a role in the destructive process: genetic, virological and immunological factors. Several arguments can be produced to support the involvement of each of these factors.

3.1. Virological etiology

Viral infections can cause diabetes mellitus (11). In humans only a few cases have been reported. In these cases hyperglycaemia and ketoacidosis developed during a severe, fatal infection with Coxsackie B4 virus. In one case the virus could be isolated from the pancreas and it produced diabetes, when it was inoculated in a strain of susceptible mice (10).

Much experimental work has been done in animals, especially in mice. The Encephalomyocarditis virus causes an acute diabetic syndrome in susceptible strains of mice within 48 hours after infection. In mice inoculated with Coxsackie B virus hyperglycaemia develops after 15-20 days. Of the Reoviruses type I is of special interest, because infection

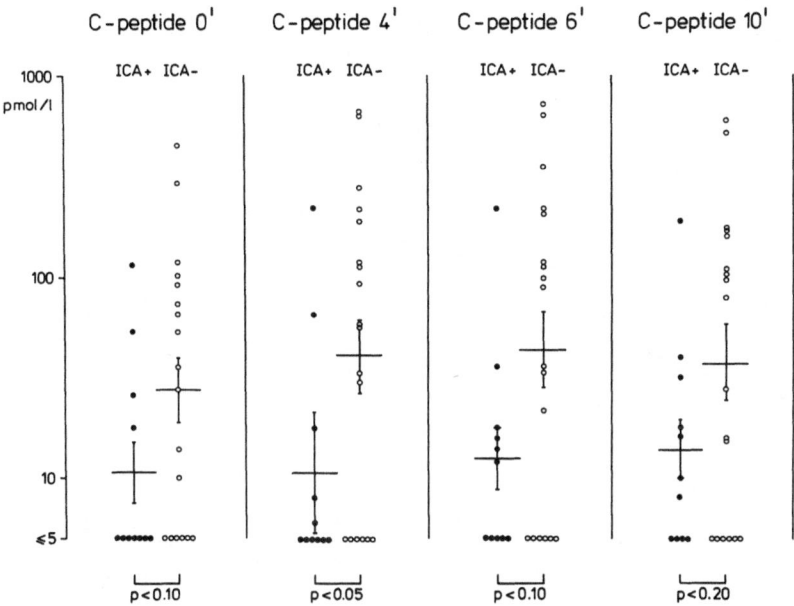

FIGURE 2. C-peptide levels in the fasting state (C-peptide 0') and 4, 6 and 10 min. after 1 mg glucagon i.v. (C-peptide 4', -6', -10', respectively) in islet cell antibody positive (ICA+) (n = 13) and negative (ICA-) (n = 22) type I diabetics 4.6 ± 1.1 years after diagnosis.

with this virus leads to a polyendocrine disease affecting at least the islets of Langerhans and the pituitary.

In a study from the group of Notkins (13) islet cell lesions were found in children with fatal viral infections. Fifty per cent of the children infected with Coxsackie B and Cytomegalovirus showed these lesions. Diabetes, however, did not develop in these children. Such lesions were found in only a few cases of rubella and varicella zoster virus infections.

A relation between mumps and type I diabetes has been suggested several times on the basis of epidemiological data. Hard evidence does not exist. However, a recent study may support such a relationship. Fifty per cent of 30 children with mumps developed ICA, but none showed signs of glucose intolerance (14).

The implication of the seasonal variation on the incidence of type I diabetes has been discussed above.

3.2. Immunological etiology

There is a clear association with other autoimmune endocrinopathies (15). About 15% of patients with idiopathic Addison's disease and 7-10% of patients with autoimmune thyroid disease have type I diabetes.

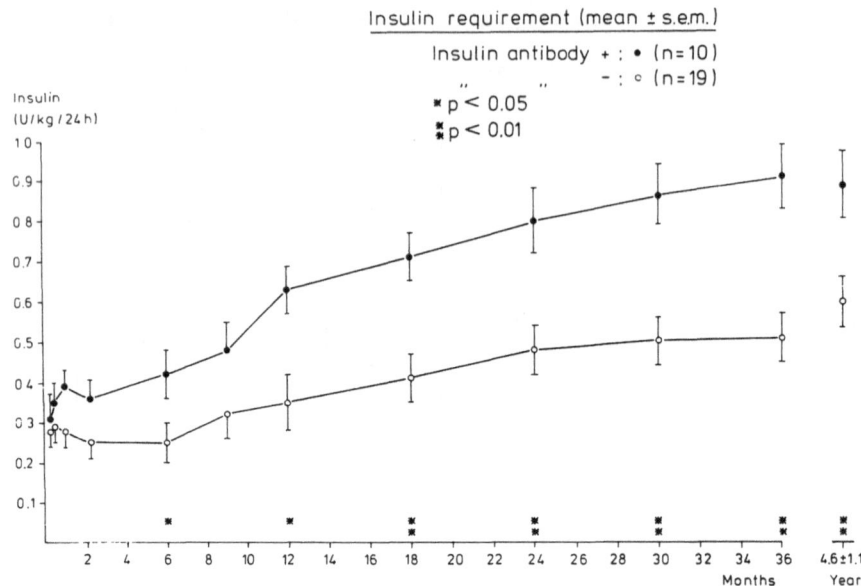

FIGURE 3. Insulin requirement (U/kg/24 h) in the first 36 months and 4.6 ± 1.1 years after diagnosis in type I diabetics who had insulin antibodies (+) (n = 10) or not (−) (n = 19) 4.6 ± 1.1 years after diagnosis.

On the other hand in type I diabetes without manifestations of other endocrine diseases about 40% have antibodies against the thyroid and/or gastric mucosa. These antibodies are mostly found in women.

Several kinds of islet cell antibodies have been detected in recent years (15). In about 60% of newly diagnosed type I diabetics cytoplasmic ICA (ICA-IgG) are found. Half of them fixes complement (CF-ICA). Islet cell surface antibodies (ICSA), directed against antigens in the cell membrane, are found in about 30% of newly diagnosed type I diabetics. CF-ICA and ICSA may be cytotoxic to B-cells.

Cell-mediated immunity also plays a role in type I diabetes. White blood cells from type I diabetics showed leucocyte migration inhibition and lymfocyte transformation with islet cell antigens (16). Changes in T-cell subpopulations have been found at the time of diagnosis. Suppressor cells may be decreased and killer cells may be increased (17).

Circulating immune complexes have been found to be elevated in newly diagnosed type I diabetics. These complexes may modulate the function of suppressor and killer cells through their Fc-IgG receptors (17).

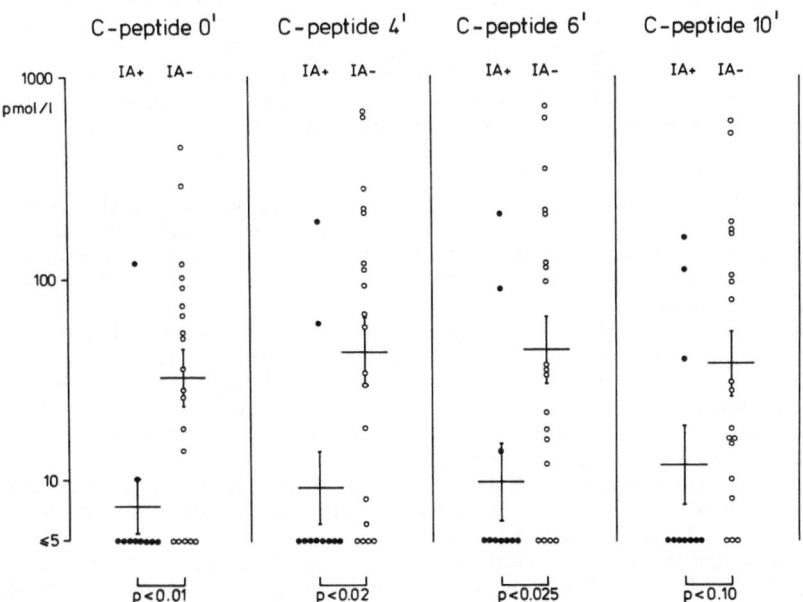

FIGURE 4. C-peptide levels in the fasting state (C-peptide 0') and 4, 6 and 10 min. after 1 mg glucagon i.v. (C-peptide 4', -6', -10', respectively) in type I diabetics with (IA+) (n = 10) and without (IA-) (n =19) insulin antibodies 4.6 ± 1.1 years after diagnosis.

Lymfocytic infiltration is often found in the islets of Langerhans within 6 months after the diagnosis of type I diabetes (18). This insulitis is specific for type I diabetes. The lymfocytes disappear from the islets in which the B-cells have been destroyed.

3.3. Genetic factors in the etiology

In studies of identical twins of which one had type I diabetes, a concordance rate for the disease of 50% has been reported (19). This means that in 50% of the twin pairs both twins had type I diabetes. In the other half of pairs one twin remained free from diabetes. This signifies that other, environmental factors must be involved in the pathogenesis of type I diabetes.

Type I diabetes is associated with antigens of the major histocompatibility complex (the HLA system in man) (20). The genetic code of this polymorphic system which for instance governs graft rejection and other immune responses is located on the short arm of the 6th chromosome. The products of these genes, the HLA antigens, are transmembrane proteins of the cell wall. More than 90% of type I diabetics are HLA-DR3 and/or -4. The highest relative risk (about 15) for type I diabetes is encountered in people who are HLA-DR3/4. Five to 10% of these will acquire the disease.

The frequency of HLA-DR3 and/or -4 in non-diabetic controls is 50-60%. Thus about half of the population may carry the genes confer- ring susceptibility to type I diabetes. However, only 0,5% or less of this population do eventually develop the disease. Therefore the ques- tion remains: Why does only one in about 100 individuals (or less) carrying one or both genes acquire type I diabetes?

The three pathogenetic factors heredity, virus infections and immuni- ty may cooperate. In susceptible subjects virus infections may pro- duce changes which induce an autoimmune reaction.

4. THERAPEUTIC PERSPECTIVE

If virological and/or immunological factors play a role in the patho- genesis of B-cell destruction, then the question could be asked, whether vaccination or immunotherapy may prevent this destruction. Vaccination is only possible, if the causative virus or viruses have been found definitely.

Ideally immunotherapy should be started when B-cell destruction begins or even earlier. At this moment it is not possible to trace exactly the beginning of B-cell destruction, although family members of type I diabetics, who share an HLA-haplotype with the proband and who are ICA positive, are at risk of developing the disease in about 50% of the cases (see above).

It may be questioned whether it is useful to start immunotherapy, when the disease has become manifest, which means that about 90% of the B-cells has been destroyed already.

At this moment such a treatment is still in the experimental stage (21, 22, 23, 24). Our knowledge on the virological and immunological genesis of type I diabetes is increasing but still fragmentary. Studies are under way which may give answers to this question (25, 26).

In the next three chapters the pathogenetic aspects of type I dia- betes will be discussed in more detail.

REFERENCES
1. Diabetes mellitus: Report of a WHO Study Group, Technical Re- port Series 727, World Health Organization, Geneva, 1985, 9.
2. Diabetes mellitus: Report of a WHO Study Group, Technical Re- port Series 727, World Health Organization, Geneva, 1985, 17-20.
3. Morrow PA, Freedman A and Craighead JE: Testosterone effect on experimental diabetes mellitus in encephalomyocarditis virus in- fected mice. Diabetologia, 18, 1980, 247-249.
4. Srikanta S, Ganda OP, Eisenbarth GS and Soeldner JS: Islet-cell antibodies and beta-cell function in monozygotic triplets and twins initially discordant for type I diabetes mellitus. New Eng J Med, 308, 1983, 322-325.
5. Srikanta S, Ganda OP, Jackson RA, Gleason RE, Kaldany A, Garovoy MR, Milford EL, Carpenter CB, Soeldner JS and Eisenbarth GS: Type I diabetes mellitus in monozygotic twins: chronic progressive beta cell dysfunction. Ann Intern Med, 99, 1983, 320-326.
6. Gorsuch AN, Lister J, Dean BM, Spencer KM, McNally JM and Bottazzo GF: Evidence for a long prediabetic period in type I (insulin-dependent) diabetes mellitus. Lancet, II, 1981, 1363-1365.
7. Spencer KM, Dean BM, Tarn A and Lister J: Fluctuating islet-cell autoimmunity in unaffected relatives of patients with insulin- dependent diabetes. Lancet, I, 1984, 764-766.

8. Bottazzo GF, Pozzilli P, Mirakian R, Dean BM and Doniach D: Early immunological events in diabetes. In: Immunology in diabetes. Andreani D, Federlin KF, Di Mario U, Heding LG. Kimpton Medical Publications, London/Edinburgh, 1984, 95-104.
9. Gamble DR: The epidemiology of insulin dependent diabetes, with particular reference to the relationship of virus infection to its etiology. Epidemiol Rev, 2, 1980, 49-70.
10. Yoon JW, Austin M, Takashi O and Notkins AL: Virus-induced diabetes mellitus: isolation of a virus from the pancreas of a child with diabetic ketoacidosis. New Eng J Med, 300, 1979, 1173-1179.
11. Toniolo A: Viruses and diabetes. In: Immunology in diabetes. Andreani D, Federlin KF, Di Mario U, Heding LG. Kimpton Medical Publications, London/Edinburgh, 1984, 71-93.
12. Barbosa J and Saner B: Do genetic factors play a role in the pathogenesis of diabetic microangiopathy? Diabetologia, 27, 1984, 487-492.
13. Jenson AB, Rosenberg HS and Notkins AL: Pancreatic islet-cell damage in children with fatal viral infections. Lancet, II, 1980, 354-358.
14. Helmke K, Otten A and Willems W: Islet cell antibodies in children with mumps infection. Lancet, II, 1980, 211-212.
15. Herold KC, Huen AHJ, Rubenstein AH and Lernmark A: Humoral abnormalities in type I (insulin-dependent) diabetes mellitus. In: Immunology in diabetes. Andreani D, Federlin KF, Di Mario U, Heding LG. Kimpton Medical Publications, London/Edinburgh, 1984, 105-120.
16. Lernmark A: Cell-mediated immunity in type I (insulin-dependent) diabetes: update 84. In: Immunology in diabetes. Andreani D, Federlin KF, Di Mario U, Heding LG. Kimpton Medical Publications, London/Edinburgh, 1984, 121-131.
17. Pozzilli P and Di Mario U: Lymphocyte subpopulations and circulating immune complexes: their relationship in the pathogenesis of type I (insulin-dependent) diabetes. In: Immunology in diabetes. Andreani D, Federlin KF, Di Mario U, Heding LG. Kimpton Medical Publications, London/Edinburgh, 1984, 133-142.
18. Gepts W: The pathology of the pancreas in human diabetes. In: Immunology in diabetes. Andreani D, Federlin KF, Di Mario U, Heding LG. Kimpton Medical Publications, London/Edinburgh, 1984, 21-34.
19. Rimoin DL and Rotter JI: The genetics of diabetes mellitus. In: Immunology in diabetes. Andreani D, Federlin KF, Di Mario U, Heding LG. Kimpton Medical Publications, London/Edinburgh, 1984, 45-62.
20. Nerup J, Christy M, Platz P, Ryder LP and Svejgaard A: Aspects of the genetics of insulin-dependent diabetes mellitus. In: Immunology in diabetes. Andreani D, Federlin KF, Di Mario U, Heding LG. Kimpton Medical Publications, London/Edinburgh, 1984, 63-70.
21. Editorial: Prevention of insulin-dependent diabetes. Lancet, I, 1983, 104-105.
22. Rossini AA: Immunotherapy for insulin-dependent diabetics? New Eng J Med, 308, 1983, 333-335.
23. Eisenbarth GS: Immunotherapy of type I diabetes. Diabetes Care, 6, 1983, 521-523.

24. Marx JL: Diabetes – a possible autoimmune disease. Science, 225, 1984, 1381–1383.
25. Stiller CR, Dupré J, Gent M, Jenner MR, Keown PA, Laupacis A, Martell R, Rodger NW, v. Graffenried B and Wolfe BMJ: Effects of cyclosporine immunosuppression in insulin-dependent diabetes mellitus of recent onset. Science, 223, 1984, 1362–1367.
26. Assan R, Debray-Sachs M, Laborie C, Chatenoud L, Feutren G, Quiniou-Debrie MC, Thomas G and Bach JF: Metabolic and immuno-logical effects of cyclosporin in recently diagnosed type 1 diabetes mellitus. Lancet, I, 1985, 67–71.

1.1.2. Autoimmune pathogenesis of viral diabetes
P.G. Babu, S.A. Huber and J.E. Graighead

Until recently, the pathogenesis of diabetes mellitus has been shrouded in confusion partly because clinicians failed to distinguish the different forms of the disease. Sense began evolving from chaos with the initial identification of two distinct entities; insulin-dependent (juvenile, type I) and insulin-independent (maturity onset, type II) diabetes mellitus. Even within this dichotomy, type I diabetes undoubtably represents a heterologous group of related diseases having distinct etiologies but ultimately resulting in destruction of the insulin producing beta cells. Autoimmunity presumably causes diabetes in patients with multiple endocrine disorders, but might additionally induce type I diabetes in most other individuals. Mononuclear cells usually infiltrate the islets of Langerhans early in the course of the disease suggesting immune mediated injury. This inflammation, termed insulitis, was observed as early as 1901 (1), but Gepts (2) is credited with the detailed description of the lesions in 1965. Two aspects of insulitis implicate it in the pathogenesis of diabetes. First, greater than 80% of patients with untreated ketonic diabetes of short duration (less than 6 months) have insulitis, and secondly, inflammation in the islets can precede beta cell loss.

The observation of insulitis alone cannot prove an immunologic etiology for type I diabetes. However, since the 1970's, additional evidence implicating autoimmunity in the disease has been reported. Originally described by Bottazzo et al (3), islet cell antibodies (ICAs) have now been found in nearly all individuals with type I diabetes either before or at the time of diagnosis (4). Nonetheless, ICAs fail to lyse cultured beta cells and react equally well with both alpha and delta cells in the islets although these cells are not affected in diabetes. While ICAs probably play no significant role in the pathogenesis of diabetes, they may function as markers for susceptibility to the disease. Pike et al (5) noted that both members of monozygotic twinships frequently developed diabetes although a considerable time may elapse between the diagnosis of the disease in the index and second sibling. During the intervening period, the unaffected sibling may generate ICAs weeks to years preceding the overt onset of hyperglycemia. The extended period between the appearance of the ICAs in these individuals and the diagnosis of diabetes further implies that these antibodies are not involved in beta cell injury. However, if diabetes susceptible individuals can produce one autoimmune antibody, they might also develop other more pathogenic autoimmune reactions. Other autoantibodies reacting specifically with beta cells arise sporadically in individuals with newly diagnosed diabetes. These antibodies, recognizing beta cell surface antigens, both lyse cultured beta cells and inhibit their metabolic function. Finally increased cellular immunity to beta cells has been reported early in the disease.

Despite the accumulating circumstantial evidence favoring an immune pathogenesis to type I diabetes mellitus, environmental factors must precipitate the disease since monozygotic twins rarely develop hyperglycemia simultaneously (6). Both chemicals and viruses have been implicated in insulin dependent diabetes clinically and experimentally (7-9). In each case, the diabetogenic agent either directly damages the beta cells or alters metabolic function. Most of the clinical evidence of a viral etiology in type I diabetes depends upon anecdotal case reports, seasonality of the disease, sero-epidemiologic associations and rare isolation of viruses at the time of diabetes diagnosis. While many viruses might cause diabetes in a small proportion of individuals, mumps, rubella and group B coxsackieviruses usually are considered likely etiologic agents (10-11).

The most striking epidemiologic characteristic favoring an infectious etiology in diabetes is its seasonality. Adams (12) first noted that nearly 85% of juvenile diabetes were diagnosed between August and April with peak incidences occurring during the summer/autumn and winter months in North America. The seasonality of the disease has now been confirmed by a number of different investigators in six countries and in both hemispheres (13-18). The seasonal clustering is most evident in younger patients with an abrupt onset of diabetic symptoms and who lacked a family history of the disease. Furthermore, Cudworth et al (19) associated the winter peak with individuals having a specific major histocompatibility antigen, HLA BW15. The clustering of diabetes during specific seasons is consistent with the hypothesis that the disease is of infectious origin since many of the suspected viruses are also most prevalent at this time.

Reports in the medical literature have variously implicated mumps, measles, chickenpox, rubella, infectious mononucleosis, influenza, coxsackieviruses and numerous unidentified agents causing acute febrile illnesses. Secondly, if a single virus was responsible for diabetes induction, one would expect considerable year-to-year variability in incidence depending upon the prevalence of the infectious agent. However, the annual variation in diabetes periodicity and incidence is remarkedly small. If many viruses can trigger the disease, annual variations in any one virus could go unnoticed.

Epidemiological studies provide additional evidence of an infectious origin to diabetes. In 1949, John (20) concluded that of 500 diabetic children in his practice, 35% had a predisposing infection prior to the onset of diabetes symptoms. Mumps was the primarily infection cited in this study, but other viruses were also obviously implicated. Other investigators have noted diabetes "epidemics" where clusters of cases occur in limited geographical areas during finite time periods. Thus, Melin and Ursing (21) found that 4 out of 42 individuals contracting mumps in a small Swedish village subsequently developed diabetes. Other examples of diabetes epidemics have been reported although a causative infectious agent has not always been identified. Finally various retrospective studies including those by Cudworth et al (19), and Gamble (13) found that between 23.9 and 39% of recently diagnosed patients gave a clinical history of a "virus-like" illness preceding the onset of diabetes.

Probably the best evidence for a viral etiology to diabetes is derived from serological and virological studies. West et al (15,22) found four-fold rises in antibody titers to coxsackieviruses in diabetic compared to control individuals. Three other investigations also demonstrated elevated coxsackievirus antibody titers in diabetic individuals, again suggesting indirectly a correlation between the viral infection and the disease. However, the best evidence that coxsackieviruses can induce diabetes came from three studies in which the virus was isolated from children simultaneously with or soon after diagnosis of diabetes. In one case the child developed ketoacidosis 3 days after the onset of a flu-like illness

(23). At autopsy, the islets showed extensive inflammatory cell infiltration. Elevated antibody titers to coxsackievirus B4 were observed and a coxsackievirus B4 was isolated from the pancreas of the patient which induced beta cell necrosis and diabetes-like disease in susceptible mice. Finally, Jenson et al (24) retrospectively studied children dying of documented viral illnesses and found that 4/7 children with fatal coxsackievirus infections also had insulitis. Inflammation was additionally observed with several other viruses, most notably with cytomegalovirus and rubella infections. Insulitis may be a relatively common result of specific viral infections.

Despite the potential of many viruses to damage beta cells, relatively few infected individuals develop overt diabetes. Susceptibility undoubtably depends upon multiple factors including the physiological state and genetics of the host. Thus, although a diabetogenic virus may exist in a population, diabetes would occur only in genetically predisposed individuals. There is clearly a genetic association between insulin dependent diabetes and the major histocompatibility antigens DR3 and DR4. This genetic region is involved in regulating immunity primarily by controlling antigen recognition. Among insulin dependent diabetics, nearly 98% have either DR antigens 3 or 4 and over half of the patients have both. Since heterozygocity for these DR antigens enhances risk of diabetes, presumably two distinct genes regulate susceptibility. Possession of either gene alone imparts some risk of the disease, but inheritance of both genes greatly accentuates the probability of contracting the disease. This was succintly demonstrated by Cudworth and Wolf (19). In families where the children could inherit DR3 and DR4, 40% of the children inherited both antigens and 81% of the heterozygous individuals ultimately developed diabetes. Furthermore, monozygotic twins were twice as likely to be concordant for diabetes when heterozygous for DR3 and DR4 than when possessing only one susceptibility antigen.

The relationship between precipitating virus infections, autoimmunity and diabetes can best be visualized in animals models of the disease. The experimental system most frequently used by investigators, including ourselves, employs the diabetogenic M variant of encephalomyocarditis (EMC-M) virus and mice. EMC-M virus is highly and rapidly lethal to cultured murine beta cells and causes hypoinsulinemia and hyperglycemia in vivo. The virus is specific for the beta cells in the islet, sparing both the alpha and delta cells and the acinar tissue (25). Presumably, the unsusceptible cells lack appropriate virus receptors on their plasma membranes preventing infection. Susceptibility to EMC-M virus induced diabetes varies strikingly among inbred strains of mice. Some investigators suggest that beta cells from diabetes resistant mice also lack virus receptors protecting the cells from infection and damage (26). This concept is controversial since other investigators including ourselves have not observed significant differences in virus attachment and concentrations between susceptible and nonsusceptible beta cells. Rather, diabetes susceptibility in mice may result from host genetic factors permitting autoimmune reactions (27).

Various immunosuppressive procedures have either partially or totally prevented the induction of diabetes in EMC-M virus infected mice. The procedures have generally been directed against the T lymphocyte, a pivotal component of immunity. Nonetheless, other investigators found no evidence for immunity in diabetes. We believe that workers implicating immunity in this disease and those opposed to this concept are both correct. The genetic constitution of the host apparently determines the pathogenic mechanisms of beta cell injury. DBA/2 and Balb/cBY mice are identical at the major histocompatibility complex of the mouse, and usually 80% or more of the animals from both strains become hyperglycemic after EMC-M virus infection. However, T lymphocyte depletion of the Balb/cBy mice significantly reduces both blood glucose levels and insulitis in infected animals while similar treatment of DBA/2 mice fails to limit the disease. The severity of hyperglycemia in DBA/2 mice directly correlates with the virus concentrations in the pancreas. Thus, diabetes in DBA/2 mice primarily results from direct virus mediated injury of the beta cells, while both virus and immune mechanisms produce the disease in Balb/cBY mice (28).

More recently, studies using another Balb/c subline, Balb/cCUM, have yielded even more intriguing results. These animals, previously considered diabetes resistant, develop a delayed and mild glucose intolerance correlating to the appearance of cytolytic T lymphocytes directed against beta cell surface antigens. Significantly, autoimmunity and glucose intolerance occur after infectious virus has disappeared from the pancreas. This model appears to resemble most closely the human disease and suggests that the virus infection modifies either the beta cell or the immune system resulting in beta cell specific autoimmunity. Future investigations must determine whether the murine model validly reflects the pathogenic mechanisms in human insulin dependent diabetes.

CONCLUDING REMARKS

Viruses might induce diabetes, but only in a proportion of affected individuals. Nonetheless, the mechanism of induction remains unclear. Our experimental work suggests that viral infection initiates autoimmune injury to the beta cells. However, extrapolation of these observations to the human disease requires further experimentation.

REFERENCES

1.   Opie EL: The relation of diabetes mellitus to lesions of the pancreas. J. Exp. Med. 5:527, 1901.
2.   Gepts W: Pathologic anatomy of the pancreas in juvenile diabetes mellitus.   Diabetes 14:619, 1965.
3.   Bottazo GF, Florin-Christensen A, Doniach D: Islet cell antibodies in diabetes mellitus with autoimmune polyendocrine deficiencies. Lancet 2:1279, 1974.
4.   Martin, Ehrlich, Holland(ed): Etiology and pathogenesis of insulin-dependent diabetes mellitus. Raven Press, New York, p. 61, 1981.
5.   Creutzfeldt (ed): The genetics of diabetes mellitus. Springer-Verlag, Berlin, p. 173, 1976.
6.   Craighead JE: Current views on the etiology of insulin-dependent diabetes mellitus. N.Engl.J.Med. 299: 1439, 1978.
7.   Karam JH, Prosser PP, LeWitt PA: Islet cell surface antibodies in a patient with diabetes mellitus after rodenticide ingestion. N.Engl.J. Med. 299:1191, 1979.
8.   Toniolo A, Onodera T, Yoon JW, Notkins AL: Induction of diabetes by cumulative environmental insults from viruses and chemicals. Nature, 288, 383, 1980.
9.   John TJ, Babu PG, Zachariah P: Dual-aetiology diabetes mellitus: a novel mouse model.   Curr.Sci.51:35, 1982.
10. Notkins AL, Yoon JW, Onodera T, Toniolo A, Jenson AB: Virus-induced diabetes mellitus. Persp.Virol.11:141, 1981.
11. Gupta S(ed): Immunology of clinical and experimental diabetes.

Plenum Medical Book Co, New York, p 295, 1984.

12. Adams SF: The seasonal variation in the onset of acute diabetes: The age of sex factors in 1000 diabetic patients. Arch.Intern.Med. 37:861, 1926.

13. Gamble DR: The epidemiology of insulin-dependent diabetes with reference to the relationship of virus infection to its etiology. Epidemiol. Rev. 2:49, 1980.

14. Christan B, Dromann H, Andersen O: Incidence, seasonal and geographical patterns of juvenile onset, insulin-dependent diabetes in Denmark. Diabetologia 13:281, 1977.

15. West R, Belmont E, Colle MP, Crepeau MP, Wilkins J, Poirier R: Epidemiologic survey of juvenile diabetes in Montreal. Diabetes 28:690,1979.

16. Sterky G, Holmgren G, Gustavson KH: The incidence of diabetes mellitus in Swedish children 1970-1975. Acta Pediatr. Scand. 67:139, 1978.

17. Durruty P, Ruiz F, Garcia de los Rios M: Age at diagnosis and seasonal variation in the onset of insulin-dependent diabetes in Chile (Southern Hemisphere). Diabetologia 17:357, 1979.

18. Krolewski AS, Warram JH: Joslin's Diabetes Mellitus. Lea and Febiger, Philadelphia, p 12, 1985.

19. Gupta S (ed): Immunology of clinical and experimental diabetes. Plenum Medical Book Co. New York, p 271, 1984.

20. John HJ: Diabetes mellitus in children. J. Pediat. 35:723, 1949.

21. Melin K and Ursing B: Diabetes mellitus som komplikation till parotitis epidemica. Nord. Med. 60:1715, 1958.

22. West R, Colle MP, Belmont E, Tangle A, Guttmann R, Hynie I, Thomas D, Wilkins J, Poirier R, Crepeau MP: Prospective study of insulin-dependent diabetes mellitus. Diabetes 30:584, 1981.

23. Yoon JW, Austin M, Onodera T, Notkins AL: Virus-induced diabetes mellitus. Isolation of a virus from the pancreas of a child with diabetic ketoacidosis. N.Engl.J.Med. 300:1173, 1979.

24. Jenson AB, Rosenberg HS, Notkins AL: Pancreatic islet cell damage in children with fatal virus infections. Lancet 2:354, 1980.

25. Craighead JE: The role of viruses in the pathogenesis of pancreatic disease and diabetes mellitus. Prog. Med. Virol. 19:161, 1975.

26. Chairez R, Yoon J, Notkins AL: Virus induced diabetes mellitus. X. Attachment of encephalomyocarditis virus and permissiveness of cultured pancreatic cells to infection. Virology 85:606, 1978.

27. Wilson GL, D'Andrea BJ, Bellomo SC, Craighead JE: Encephalomyocarditis virus infection of cultured murine pancreatic B cells. Nature 285, 112, 1980.

28. Huber SA, Babu PG, Craighead JE: (unpublished observations).

1.1.3. Immunological features of insulin-dependent diabetes mellitus
F. Becker and G.F. Bottazzo

INTRODUCTION

The past decade has witnessed tremendous advances in our understanding of the role that a variety of immunological processes may play in initiating and sustaining damage to pancreatic Beta cells.

The most exciting development in recent years has been the demonstration that, despite the acute onset of clinical symptoms, the disease results from long, slow and progressive damage to the pancreatic Beta cells (1). This evidence was obtained primarily by the study of unaffected first degree relatives of patients with childhood diabetes (2). At the same time it was shown that siblings who shared one or two HLA-haplotypes with the diabetic proband had a greatly increased risk of developing the disease (3). These genetic markers and the presence of a variety of islet cell antibodies (ICA) identify potential candidates for Type 1 diabetes with a reasonably high degree of precision.

HUMORAL IMMUNITY
Islet-cell antibodies (ICA)

ICA are organ specific for endocrine pancreas, they cross-react with other species and are of IgG class. Several antigens including some that are only present in beta cells are now envisaged in what is basically a polyclonal autoimmune response with subclass restrictions (4). The antibodies may be complement fixing (CF-ICA) and this is a separate variant (5). The more common islet-cell antibodies are not able to fix complement (ICA-IgG). As the islet-cell antigens have not yet been isolated and are at present only partially characterized (6) cytoplasmic ICA are normally detected by standard immunofluorescence (IFL). Unfixed blood group O human pancreas is still the substrate of choice (7). Fixed pancreas substrates give controversial readings, especially in complement-fixation immunofluorescence tests with anti-C3 conjugates used to detect CF-ICA (8).

In the screening test ICA-IgG reacts with all four endocrine cells (9). This 'shared' autoantigen is not represented on the cell surface and therefore cannot be in direct contact with sensitized lymphocytes in the living gland. Since circulating antibodies exert cytotoxic effects through complement-dependent mechanisms, extensive parallel tests for ICA-IgG and CF-ICA revealed that in almost all diabetic groups tested, only half the islet-cell antibodies fixed complement (5). Most significantly, this was also found in genetically predisposed first-degree relatives who later became diabetic. This percentage was only higher (75%) in 'polyendocrine' patients positive for ICA but not diabetic (10). This led to the conclusion that CF-ICA reactions include the beta-cell-specific autoantibodies that are the most relevant markers for ongoing insulitis. We now know that some CF-ICA selectively stain beta cells (11). We also found some sera containing complement-fixing variants specific for glucagon or somatostatin cells. These single-cell antibodies were known to exist in some diabetic sera (12).

Islet-cell surface antibodies (ICSA)

ICSA would certainly appear to have greater pathogenic significance than ICA, since they represent the initial attack on the plasma membrane of viable Beta cells. At present, however, ICA retains its usefulness for routine screening.

ICSA are detected by fluorescence or Staphylococcus Aureus protein A techniques on viable cultured human foetal (13) or adult animal pancreas (14). Since human sera contain heterophile antibodies which stain animal pancreas non-specifically, despite prolonged absorption with other animal tissues, human islets (although hard to obtain) remain the tissue of choice. In both human and animal tissue diabetic sera contain separate specificities for Beta and to a lesser extent Alpha and Delta cells. Using a cell sorter technique to separate the ICSA positive cells (15) a small number of sera were identified containing surface reacting antibodies to pancreatic polypeptide (PP) cells. Antibodies to these cells have not as yet been detected on cryostat sections, probably because it is necessary to employ the mid-posterior portion of the head of the pancreas, which is known to be rich in PP cells (16).

A high proportion of newly diagnosed diabetic sera contain ICSA, but about 30% give negative results on sections (14). This suggests the involvement of an additional antigen that is expressed entirely on the plasma membrane of Beta cells. ICSA tend to disappear in the course of time like other autoimmune phenomena in Type I diabetes.

They have cytotoxic effects 'in vitro', when fresh complement is added to the culture medium. The lysing effect is preferentially against insulin cells as assessed using vital dyes (17) or the ^{51}Chromium release assay (18). Immunoglobulin preparations obtained from ICSA positive sera produced significant inhibition of glucose induced insulin release when isolated rat islet cells were incubated for a short period without the addition of complement (19). It has been claimed that when whole islets separated from human (20) or animal (21) pancreas are incubated with diabetic sera, repeated addition of complement over 18 hours also resulted in potent inhibition of insulin secretion. Arginine-stimulated glucagon release remained unchanged. The role of complement, either in exerting direct cytotoxic effects or by enhancing blockade of secretion mechanisms by ICSA, has yet to be clarified (22). In all experiments of this type it is highly advisable to check islet cell viability when experiments are performed in the presence of complement.

In selected sera it has been found that certain ICSA do not exert complement dependent cytotoxicity, but rather have a potent lytic effect in an antibody-dependent cell mediated cytotoxicity (ADCC) system. This primarily involves killer (K) lymphocytes (23).

Anti-insulin- and anti-insulin receptor antibodies

The spontaneous development of insulin autoantibodies is becoming increasingly important within the context of pancreatic autoimmunity. The full 'insulin autoimmune syndrome' is mainly seen in Japan (24) but exists in other countries to a lesser extent (25). The patients, most of whom had thyrotoxicosis treated with methimazole, present with attacks of hypoglycaemia which may recur over months but with a tendency to spontaneous remission. Insulin antibodies have also been described in newly diagnosed patients with Type I diabetes (26) and in some non-diabetic polyendocrine cases (27). Related to this interesting finding is the description of insulin receptor antibodies of the IgM class in untreated juvenile diabetic patients (28). Until now IgG anti-insulin receptor antibodies were associated with a rare form of diabetes characterised by extreme insulin resistance and associated with acanthosis nigricians (29). The antibodies in the diabetic children were able to displace radioactive insulin from its receptors and also stimulated adipocyte metabolism. Although this work needs confirmation in view of the known binding to, and effects on function of the Fc fragment from normal immunoglobulins on adipocytes binding and function (30), one wonders if these receptor antibodies are secondary to the spontaneous insulin autoimmunization. The presence of these two types of autoimmune reaction suggests that insulin may act as a powerful immunogen, especially if inappropriate secretion of immature molecules occurs during the slow process of autoimmune Beta cell damage (31).

CELL MEDIATED IMMUNITY (CMI)

Our understanding of the role of cell mediated immunity in the pathogenesis of Type I diabetes has progressed slowly when compared with the rapidity of developments in the field of pancreatic humoral autoimmunity. There are several possible reasons for this. CMI techniques are much more laborious and lack the precision needed to dissect such an heterogeneous cell population. Basic immunology is still struggling in its attempt to define the physiological mechanisms underlying this arm of the immune system. Even the monoclonal antibody revolution has not helped to clarify this issue. With these reagents it is now possible to identify various subsets of lymphocytes and other immune cells (32). Even so, studies with the specific aim of detecting abnormalities of lymphocyte subpopulations at the time of diagnosis have failed to reach significant conclusions (reviewed in 33). Disagreement mainly concerns the total number of T lymphocytes, helper and cytotoxic/suppressor lymphocytes in newly diagnosed diabetic patients. Another important factor, often underestimated, is the effect on the immune system of the profound metabolic derangement produced by the disease itself (34).

The most consistent results have been obtained by measurement of 'activated' T cells at the time of diagnosis (35, 36). Here again, these tend to re-enter the normal range within months of starting on insulin therapy (37). T cells, when stimulated by antigens, express new surface markers which are essential for an efficient participation in the immune response. The present hypothesis is that T cells are activated in diabetes because they have been stimulated specifically by pancreatic antigens, and not just triggerred by environmental agents.

GENETICS

The total genetic contribution cannot exceed 50% since this is the maximum estimate of the rate of concordance in identical twins with Type 1 diabetes. Different haplotypes in the major histocompatibility complex are now implicated, involving HLA-DR3, DR4 and several 'complotypes', i.e. allotypes of the complement components C2, C4 and Bf. This entire set of genes on Chrosome 6 has been calculated to account for between 60 and 70% of the genetic susceptibility. This leaves another 30-40% of the risk to be accounted for by genes on other chromosomes (38). The present candidates include Chromosome 11 where DNA sequences flanking the insulin gene probably contribute to susceptibility (39,40) and Chromosome 14 where the immunoglobin heavy chain genes are situated. There is controversy as to whether Ig heavy chain genes do or do not contribute to Type I diabetes, but there is some evidence that they are involved in susceptibility to Graves' disease (41). Another candidate is Chromosome 2 which contains the kappa light chain immunoglobulin genes, and genes for the blood groups Lewis and Kidd (42). It has been found that one of the haplotypes of the Kappa light chain constant region (Kml) was over-represented in affected as against non-affected siblings (43). Because of the close association between genes coding for the constant and variable regions of immunoglobulins (there are no genetic markers for the latter in human beings), this study concluded that the putative diabetogenic genes were coded in the V region. Lambda chain genes could not be examined because the corresponding allotypic markers are not available and no correlation was observed with Gm groups in family studies. Although this hypothesis has great potential interest, both the analysis of the raw data in this paper and the conclusions reached have been questioned (44). The same applies to the association between diabetes and Kidd blood group genotype (45).

ABERRANT HLA-DR EXPRESSION

The Class II histocompatibility molecules encoded by genes in the HLA-D region play a key role in the presentation of antigens and regulation of the immune response. The expression of these cell surface glycoproteins is normally restricted to B-lymphocytes, macrophages, dendritic and other antigen presenting cells and capillary endothelium (46). Modulation of HLA-DR expression has been observed only exceptionally outside the immune system. Thus, guinea pig mammary gland, duct and epithelium become Ia positive during pregnancy and lactation (47). Expression of Class II molecules can be induced during graft-versus-host disease (48) and in some forms of cancer (49).

Our own recent hypothesis concerning the generation of organ-specific autoimmunity (50) was based on the observation that DR antigen expression could be induced in normal thyroid cells (51) and that DR glycoproteins were spontaneously expressed on thyrocytes of glands from patients with thyrotoxicosis or Hashimoto's thyroiditis (52). These findings have been extended to the pancreatic B-cell in the context of diabetic insulitis (53). Similar data have recently been obtained in biopsies from patients with primary biliary cirrhosis (54) and alopecia areata (55), conditions thought to have an autoimmune etiology.

The new hypothesis envisages the following series of events. Viruses or other environmental agents present in the endocrine tissues of genetically predisposed individuals do not necessarily confer signs of overt infection, nor do they need to be strictly organ-specific. These factors could enhance the production of gamma-interferon, a known inducer of HLA-DR expression (56). The aberrant expression of DR molecules on endocrine glands leads to the correct presentation of surface autoantigens and subsequent induction of autoreactive T-cells. These T-cells would in turn produce more interferon, maintaining DR molecular production and expression on the target organ and activation of effector B- and T-lymphocytes. Whether the initial activation of autoreactive T-cells leads to autoimmune disease would depend on a variety of other factors such as selective abnormalities of the suppressor T-cell pathway reported to coexist with autoimmunity (57).

CONSIDERATIONS AND FUTURE TRENDS

Enviromental factors remain elusive. Suggested agents are in any case common in the population, and may have exerted their effects years before the onset of the clinical condition. We cannot rule out the possibility, however, that they may have a synergistic effect in genetically susceptible individuals in whom the process of Beta cell destruction is already under way.

Autoimmunity appears to be more important in the slow process of Beta cell destruction. Whether primary or secondary, autoimmune processes are at least demonstrable, subject to a variety of laboratory tests, and capable of careful dissection and characterization.

A few years ago the division into Type I or insulin-dependent (IDDM) and Type II or non-insulin-dependent diabetes (NIDDM) helped to overcome the problem of age at onset, when it was realized that IDDM could occur at any age and that at least 2 genetic subspecies of NIDDM existed in young people (MODY). In considering IDDM itself, it was thought for some time already that 'polyendocrine' or 'autoimmune' IDDM could be clearly distinguished from the more common juvenile onset cases (58). The immunofluorescent serological markers made it possible to examine large numbers of patients and to separate Type I diabetes from all milder forms of the disease. There is general agreement that about 10% of Type I diabetics present many of the characteristics of 'primary' endocrine autoimmune disorders (Table 1). In the other 90%, IDDM usually starts in childhood, there is a 12-20% male excess and seasonal variations as well as considerable ethnic differences. In children the disappearance of the pancreatic autoimmune markers down to 20% between 3 to 5 years after clinical onset is still puzzling. This applies, as stated previously, to all types of ICA, to the cell mediated pancreatic immunity, to the mononuclear cell infiltration in the pancreas, and to some of the anomalies of T lymphocyte subsets including DR-positive 'activated' T-cells. It is considered that the two subsets of IDDM Types 1a and 1b and the insulitis are triggered by combinations of environmental insults and genetic predisposition to organ-specific autoimmunity centred on the endocrine pancreas (10).

Effort should now be concentrated on developing techniques to 'immortalise' pancreatic Beta cells. When available in large quantities these may prove an invaluable means of devising new methods (such as RIA and ELISA) for ICA determination. These could then be used to screen large populations. In addition the availability of islet cells in adequate numbers is an essential pre-requisite for expanding Beta cell specific T-cell clones, as it has recently been demonstrated for autoimmune thyroid disease (59). This might open the way to selective therapeutic intervention (60). Levels of 'activated' T cells need to be measured systematically at the time of diagnosis and most important, prospectively in 'high risk' individuals. T cells expressing IL-2 - the T cell growth factor receptor (another marker of T cell activation) - will be the most suitable cells for subsequent cloning.

It is imperative to produce monoclonal antibodies recognizing relevant epitopes on islet cells. These reagents would offer another important tool for the purification of Beta cell autoantigen(s). With this technique we would also be in an ideal position for fusing

B lymphocytes from ICA positive pre-diabetic individuals in order to monitor the subsequent destruction of Beta cells in a prospective manner, and to define those specificities more closely related to onset of the disease.

At the onset of clinical diabetes, 80-90% of beta-cells have lost the capacity to secrete insulin and it is too late to detect differences in the pathogenetic mechanisms between one subgroup of the same disease and another. To find out the sequence of events it is necessary to study susceptible individuals in the latency period.

It is very much on the cards that islets may regenerate especially during the long latency period, and involvement of hormones from other endocrine glands or distinct immunological factors in the putative regenerative process remains an attractive possibility.

TABLE 1.   DISTINCTIVE FEATURES OF 'JUVENILE ONSET' (Ia) VERSUS
'POLYENDOCRINE' (Ib) INSULIN–DEPENDENT DIABETES MELLITUS

Features	Type Ia	Type Ib
% of total IDDM population	80–90%	10–20%
Insulin requirement	Obligatory	Sometimes delayed
Residual beta–cell function	Low to absent	Often low normal
Clinical features at onset	Severe	Often less severe
'Honeymoon' period	Short	Not known
Seasonal variation	Yes	No
Sex ratio male/female	1.2/1	1/3
Age at onset of symptoms	Peak: 10–14 years	Any age, mainly adults
Associated autoimmune disorders	Unusual	Frequent
Prevalence of other autoantibodies	Low	High
Presence of ICA:		
at onset	60–85%	Not known
after 1 year	40%	42%
after 5 years	15–20%	
CF–ICA as % of total ICA	50%	66% – 75%
Appearence of ICA	Years before the onset of symptoms	Years before the onset of symptoms
Fluctuation of ICA	ICA reappeared in 27% of diabetics after 5–20 years	Tend to persist

REFERENCES

1. Bottazzo GF, Pozzilli P, Mirakian R, Dean BM, Doniach D (1984): Early imunological events in diabetes. In: Immunology in Diabetes, Chapter 7, pp. 95-104. Editors: D. Andreani, U. Di Mario, K.F. Federlin and L.G. Heding. Kimpton, London.
2. Gorsuch AN, Spencer KM, Lister J, McNally JM, Dean BM, Bottazzo GF, Cudworth AG (1981): The natural history of Type 1 (insulin-dependent) diabetes mellitus: evidence for a long pre-diabetic period. Lancet, 2, 136 1363-1365.
3. Gorsuch AN, Spencer KM, Lister J, Wolf E, Bottazzo GF, Cudworth AG (1982): Can future Type 1 diabetes be predicted? A prospective study in families of affected children. Diabetes, 31, 862-866.
4. Dean BM, Bottazzo GF, Cudworth AG (1983): IgG subclass distribution in organ-specific autoantibodies. The relationship to complement fixing ability. Clin. Exp. Immunol. 52, 61-66.
5. Bottazzo GF, Dean BM, Gorsuch AN, Cudworth AG, Doniach D (1980): Complement-fixing islet cell antibodies in Type I Diabetes: Possible monitors of active beta-cell damage. Lancet, 1, 668-672.
6. Baekkeskov S, Nielsen JH, Marner B, Bilde T, Ludvigsson J, Lernmark A (1982): Autoantibodies in newly diagnosed diabetic children immunoprecipitate human pancreatic islet cell proteins. Nature (London), 298, 167-169.
7. Bottazzo GF, Florin-Christensen A, Doniach D (1974): Islet cell antibodies in diabetes mellitus with autoimmune polyendocrine deficiency. Lancet, 2, 1279-1283.
8. Dean B, Pujol-Borrell R, Bottazzo GF (1982): Determination of islet cell antibodies by immunofluorescence. (Letter to the Editor) Lancet 2, 1343-1344.
9. Bottazzo GF, Doniach D (1978): Islet-cell antibodies in diabetes mellitus. Evidence of an autoantigen common to all cells in the islets of Langerhans. Ric. clin. Labor., 8, 29-38.
10. Becker F, Tarn AC, Gale EAM, Doniach D, Bottazo GF (1985): In search of heterogeneity in the pre-diabetic period. In: Proceedings of the 6th International Beilinson Symposium on Future Trends in Juvenile Diabetes. Z Laron and M Karp (Eds). S Karger, Basel (in press)
11. Bottazzo GF, Mirakian R, Dean BM, McNally JM, Doniach D (1982): How immunology helps to define heterogeneity in diabetes mellitus. In: The Genetics of Diabetes Mellitus, pp 79-90. Editors: J. Kobberling and R Tattersall. Academic Press, London.
12. Bottazzo GF, Lendrum R (1976): Separate autoantibodies to human pancreatic glucagon and somatostatin cells. Lancet 2, 873-876.
13. Pujol-Borrell R, Khoury EL, Bottazzo GF (1982): Islet cell surfae antibodies in Type I (insulin-dependent) diabetes mellitus: use of human fetal pancreas cultures as substrate. Diabetologia, 22, 89-95.
14. Papadopoulos GK, Lernmark A (1983): The spectrum of islet cell antibodies. In: Autoimmune Endocrine Disease, pp. 167-180. Editor: TF Davies, John Wiley, New York.
15. Van de Winkel M, Smets G, Gepts W, Pipeleers D (1982): Islet cell surface antibodies from insulin-dependent diabetics bind specifically to pancreatic B cells. J. Clin. Invest. 70, 41-49.

16. Orci L (1982): Macro- and micro-domains in the endocrine pancreas. Diabetes, 31, 538–565.
17. Dobersen MJ, Schaff JE, Ginsberg-Fellner F, Notkins, AL (1982): Preferential lysis of Beta cells by islet cell surface antibodies. Diabetes, 31, 459–462.
18. Kanatsuna T, Freedman ZR, Rubenstein AH, Lernmark A (1982): Effect of islet cell surface antibodies and complement on the release of insulin and chromium from perifused Beta cells. Clin. Exp. Immunol., 47, 85–92.
19. Kanatsuna T, Baekkeskov S, Lernmark A, Ludvigsson J (1983): Immunoglobulin from insulin dependent diabetic children inhibits glucose induced insulin release. Diabetes, 32, 520–524.
20. Sai P, Boitard Chr, Debray-Sachs M, Pouplard A, Assan R, Hamburger J (1981): Complement fixing islet cell antibodies from some diabetic patients alter insulin release in vitro. Diabetes, 30, 1051–1057.
21. Boitard C, Sai P, Debray-Sachs M, Assan R, Hamburger J (1984): Anti-pancreatic immunity. In vitro studies of cellular and humoral immune reactions directed toward pancreatic islets. Clin. Exp. Immunol. 55, 571–580.
22. Debray-Sachs M, Quiniou MC, Assan R, Bach JF (1984): Correlation between complement dependent cytotoxic and insulin release inhibitory antibodies to Beta cells in the serum of patients with IDDM. In: Immunology in Diabetes '84 p. 33. Editor: M Iavocoli. Novo Farmaceutica-Italia, Rome.
23. Marayuma T, Takei I, Matsuba I, Tsuruoka A, Taniyama M, Ikeda Y, Kataoka K, Abe M, Matsuki S (1984): Cell-mediated cytotoxic islet cell surface antibodies to human pancreatic Beta cell. Diabetologia, 26 30–33.
24. Hirata Y (1983): Methimazole and insulin autoimmune syndrome with hypoglycaemia. (Letter to the Editor) Lancet, 2 1037–1038.
25. Burden AC, Rosenthal FD (1983): Methimazole and insulin autoimmune syndrome. (Letter to the Editor) Lancet, 2, 311.
26. Palmer JP, Asplin CM, Clemons P, Lyen K, Tatpati O, Raghu PK, Paquette TL (1983): Insulin antibodies in insulin-dependent diabetics before insulin treatment. Science, 222 1337–1339.
27. Wilkin J, Nicholson S (1984): Autoantibodies against human insulin. Br. Med. J., 288 349–352.
28. Maron R, Elias D, Jongh BM, Bruining GJ, Van Rood JJ, Schechter Y, Cohen IR (1983): Autoantibodies to the insulin receptor in juvenile onset of insulin dependent diabetes. Nature (London), 817–818.
29. Kahn CR, Kasuga M, King GS, Grunfeld C (1982): Autoantibodies to insulin receptors in man: immunological determinants and mechanisms of action. In: Receptor Antibodies and Disease Ciba Symposium 90, pp 91–106. Pitman, London.
30. Khoker MA, Dandona P (1983): Insulin-like stimulatory effect of Fc fragments of human immunoglobulin G on rat adipocyte lipogenesis: indirect evidence for Fc receptor on adipocytes. J. Clin. Endocrinol. Metab., 56 393–396.
31. Rotter JI, Rimoin DL (1983): Genetics of Type I diabetes. Acta Endocrinol. (Copenhagen), 103, suppl. 256 26A.
32. Bernard A, Bounsell L, Dausset J, Milstein C, Schlossman SF (Eds) (1984): Leucocyte Typing. Springer-Verlag, Berlin.

33. Bottazzo GF, Pujol-Borrell R, Gale E (1985): Etiology of diabetes: the role of autoimmune mechanisms. In: 'The Diabetes Annual/I' p.16-52. KGMM Alberti and LP Krall (eds). Elsevier Science Publ. Amsterdam.
34. Rodier M, Andary M, Richard JL, Mirouze J, Clot J (1984): Peripheral blood T-cell subsets studied by monoclonal antibodies in Type I (Insulin-dependent) diabetes: effect of blood glucose control. Diabetologia, 27, Suppl., 136-138.
35. Jackson RA, Morris MA, Haynes BF, Eisenbarth GS (1982): Increased circulating Ia antigen-bearing T cells in Type I diabetes mellitus. N. Engl. J. Med., 306, 785-788.
36. Pozzilli P, Zuccarini O, Iavicoli M, Andreani D, Sensi M, Spencer KM, Bottazzo GF, Beverley PCL, Kyner JL, Cudworth AG (1983): Monoclonal antibodies defined abnormalities of T lymphocytes in Type I (insulin-dependent) diabetes. Diabetes, 32, p. 91-94.
37. Alviggi L, Johnston C, Hoskins DJ, Tee DEH, Pyke D, Leslie RDG, Vergann D (1984): Pathogenesis of insulin-dependent diabetes: a role for activated T lymphocytes. Lancet, 2, 4-6.
38. Bottazzo GF, Todd I, Pujol-Borrell R (1984): Hypothesis for the genetic contributions to the aetiology of diabetes mellitus. Immunol. Today. 5, 230-231.
39. Bell GI, Horita S, Karam JN (1984): A polymorphic locus near the human insulin genes is associated with insulin-dependent diabetes mellitus. Diabetes, 33, 176-183.
40. Hitman GA, Tarn AC, Drummond V, Williams LG, Joweti NI, Bottazzo GF, Galton DJ (1985): An association of insulin-dependent diabetes with a highly variable locus close to the insulin gene on chromosome 11. Diabetologia, 28, 218-222.
41. Bothwell A (1983): Enhancement, translocation and the behaviour of V genes. Immunol. Today, 4, 315.
42. Hodge SE, Anderson OE, Neis-Wanger K, Spencer MA, Sparkes RS, Sparkes MC, Crist M, Terasaki PI, Rimoin DL, Rotter JL (1981): Close genetic linkage between diabetes mellitus and kidd blood group. Lancet, 2, 893-895.
43. Adams DD, Adams YJ, Knight JG, McCall J White P, Horrocks R, Loghem E (1984): A solution to the genetic and environmental puzzles of insulin-dependent diabetes mellitus. Lancet, 1, 420-423.
44. Field LL, Anderson CE, Rimoin DL (1984): Inheritance of immunoglobulin light chain genes in pairs of siblings with insulin dependent diabetes mellitus. (Letter to the Editor) Lancet 1, 1132.
45. Barbosa J, Chavers B, Dunsworth T, Michael A (1982): Islet cell antibodies and histocompatibility antigens in insulin-dependent diabetics and their first degree relatives. Diabetes, 31, 585-588.
46. Barclay AN, Mason DW (1982): Induction of Ia antigen in rat epidermal cells and gut epithelium by immunological stimuli. J. Exp. Med., 156, 1665-1676.
47. Klareskog L, Forsum U, Peterson PA (1980): Hormonal regulation of the expression of I antigens on mammary gland epithelium. Eur. J. Immunol., 10, 958-963.
48. Barclay AN, Mason DW (1983): Graft rejection and Ia antigens - paradox resolved? Nature (London), 303, 382-383.
49. Lloyd KO, Ng J, Diffold WG (1981): Analysis of the biosynthesis of HLA-DR glycoproteins in human malignant melanoma cell lines. J. Immunol., 126, 2408-2413.

50. Bottazzo GF, Pujol-Borrell R, Hanafusa T, Feldmann M (1983): Hypothesis: role of aberrant HLA-DR expression and antigen presentation in the inductions of endocrine autoimmunity. Lancet, 2,, 1115-1119.

51. Pujol-Borrell R, Hanafusa T, Chiovata L, Bottazzo GF (1983): Lectin-induced expression of DR antigen on human cultured follicular thyroid cells. Nature (London), 304, 71-73.

52. Hanafusa T, Pujol-Borrell R, Chiovata L, Russell RCG, Doniach D, Bottazzo GF (1983): Aberrant expression of HLA-DR antigen on thyrocytes in Graves' disese: relevance for autoimmunity. Lancet, 2, 1111-1115.

53. Bottazzo GF, Dean BM (1984): Evidence of the expression of Class II (HLA-DR) and increased presentation of Class I (HLA-A,B,C) molecules in pancreatic islets in Type I (insulin-dependent) diabetes, Diabetologia, 27, 259A.

54. Ballardini G, Bianchi F, Mirakian R, Pisi E, Doniach D, Bottazzo GF (1984): Aberrant expression of HLA-DR antigens on bile duct epithelium in primary biliary cirrhosis: relevance to pathogenesis. Lancet ii, 1009-1013.

55. Messenger AG, Bleehen SS, Slater DN, Rooney N (1984): Expression of HLA-DR in hair follicles in allopecia areata. Lancet, 2, 287.

56. Todd I, Pujol-Borrell R, Hammond L, Bottazzo GF, Feldmann M (1985): Interferon-gamma induces HLA-DR expression by thyroid epithelium. Clin. Exp. Immunol. 61, 265-273.

57. Topliss D, How T, Lewis H, Row V, Volpe R (1983): Evidence of cell-mediated immunity and specific function in Grave's disease and diabetes mellitus. J. Clin. Endocrinol. Metabol., 57, 700-705.

58. Bottazzo GF, Pujol-Borrell R, Doniach D (1981): Humoral and cellular immunity in Diabetes Mellitus. Clin. Immunol. Allergy 1, 63-80.

59. Londei M, Bottazzo GF, Feldmann M. (1985): Human T-cell clones from autoimmune thyroid glands: specific recognition of autologous thyroid cells. Science 228 p. 85-88.

60. Bottazzo GF (1984): B-cell damage in diabetic insulitis: are we approaching the solution? Diabetologia, 26, 241-249.

1.1.4. Genetic counselling in Diabetes Mellitus
R.B. Tattersall

1. INTRODUCTION

My impression (probably wrong) is that professional genetics are more often asked to advise about rare but serious diseases, especially those with onset in infancy, than about common conditions like diabetes with a variable, and usually later, age of onset. If the disease in question has simple Mendelian inheritance and full penetrance, risk calculation is straightforward. For example, if a parent has Huntington's chorea (autosomal dominant) the risk to any child is 1:2. If "healthy" parents have an infant with phenylketonuria (autosomal recessive) the chance of future children being effected is 1:4. If a boy develops haemophilia (sex linked recessive), his male siblings have a 1:2 risk while all his sisters will be carriers. These single gene disorders have the further characteristic that many can be diagnosed prenatally and the birth of affected children prevented.

Diabetes has long been known as "the geneticics nightmare" and partly for this reason and because it is so common, professional genetics have given it a wide berth. However, one could also argue that professional genetic counselling is not appropriate in diabetes because of the general rule (1) that as the genetics become progressively more obscure, so the empirical risks lessen. It is simple uncomplicated transmission that gives the really bad chances such as 1:2 or 1:4. A further consideration is that the advice given to a diabetic patient depends heavily on non-genetic considerations which only the physician can assess. Hence, I agree that the diabetologist should take the role of genetic counsellor to his patients.

2. MAKING A DIAGNOSIS

The essential first step in genetic counselling is to make as accurate a diagnosis as possible. The diagnosis of hyperglycaemia is, of course, straightforward although its cause is often less so.

Diabetes is a very heterogeneous disorder with potentially a wide variety of pathogenetic mechanisms; these range from the purely environmental, through partially genetic, to totally genetic. Known environmental causes include drugs such as steroids, Diazoxide, L-Asparaginase and probably even diuretics and beta blockers (2). Other acquired causes of hyperglycaemia, such as acromegaly and chronic pancreatitis, may escape detection in the busy diabetic clinic. From the point of view of genetic counselling, the foregoing conditions are important since there is no inherited risk. It should not be forgotten that at least 30 distinct inherited conditions are associated with diabetes (3) and will only be recognised by those who know their existence and are on the lookout for them. Certain types of diabetes do have Mendelian inheritance; the DIDMOAD (Diabetes Insipidus, Diabetes Mellitus, Optic Atrophy and Deafness) syndrome is autosomal recessive while Maturity Onset type Diabetes of the Young (MODY) is dominant (4). These rare conditions probably account for less than 1% of the totality of diabetes. The other 99% of cases, although most certainly heterogeneous, are termed "idiopathic" and divided on clinical grounds into type I (insulin dependent) and type II (insulin independent). This distinction, which is crucial for genetic counselling, is by no means as clear cut or easy to make as is sometimes implied (5). Important clinical criteria for recognising insulin dependent diabetes (IDDM) at any age are ketonuria, low body weight, substantial weight loss and severe symptoms. C-peptide measurements, HLA typing and islet cell antibodies are useful confirmatory tests but are not widely available. For the purpose of genetic counselling, it is probably safe to assume that any patient with a "classical" onset started on insulin by a competant physician has IDDM (6).

3. HOW MUCH AND WHAT SHOULD A PATIENT BE TOLD?

In surgery a doctor has a duty to warn his patient about the foreseeable risks of treatment and the same principle of full disclosure should apply with equal force to genetic counselling. In English and American law there is one exception to the above in that the doctor has a "therapeutic privilege" to withold information if it is thought that disclosure would have a serious psychological effect on the patient. In genetic counselling this exception should be used extremely sparingly. It is debatable whether a doctor should foist genetic counselling on a patient who does not specifically ask for it and yet, one knows that many patients do not ask because they fear the answer. In fact, their fears are often exaggerated since the old wives' tales which are their only source of information seldom err on the side of optimism.

Giving genetic advice involves much more than the assessment of risks and quoting of chances. Much can be done to dispel feelings of guilt and to demolish old wives' tales. Patients can be helped to rationalise their problems, to live with the hard lot that may be theirs, to reconcile themselves to deprivation or realistically face a measure of risk.

4. INSULIN DEPENDENT DIABETES

One of the commonest scenarios is the following: a 25 year old woman with IDDM has just got married and comes with her healthy husband. There is no other history of diabetes on either side of the family. The questions which this couple are like to ask are:
1. What are the risks to the mother during pregnancy?
2. What are the short term risks to the foetus?
3. What are the long term risks of the baby developing diabetes?
4. What of the mother's long term health?
5. Is there any possibility that diabetes can be cured in the mother or prevented in the baby?

4.1. Risks to the mother during pregnancy

The risk of death is very little, if any, different from that for any other pregnant women. Twenty years ago it was standard practise to admit pregnant diabetic women to hospital for most or all of the last trimester for bed rest and "meticulous" blood glucose control. With home blood glucose monitoring near normoglycaemia can be achieved and documented as an outpatient and in our unit the mean hospital stay from conception to delivery is now nine days (7). The main indication for longer hospitalisation than the average is pre-eclampsia which is more common in diabetic women in general (8) and virtually certain if the woman either has diagnosed hypertension or persistent proteinuria before pregnancy. The diabetic woman is also much more likely than her non-diabetic sister to have a caesarian section; in many units in Europe and North America the section rate runs between 50 and 60% (7).

Whether pregnancy influences the spontaneous course of micro-vascular complications, particularly retinopathy, is still not known. Several recent papers suggest the following conclusions: the spontane-ous course of retinopathy is influenced by pregnancy. Deterioration is seen in about 20% of women with background retinopathy although regression is common at delivery. Proliferative retinopathy is associated with increased obstetric complications and a worse foetal outcome. The development of proliferative retinopathy during pregnancy is not an indication for termination but will require photocoagulation (9-11).

4.2. Short term risks to the foetus

During the past 40 years peri-natal mortality of infants of diabetic women has fallen from 40% to less than 4% in most specialist units. Neo-natal complications such as macrosomia, respiratory distress syndrome, hypoglycaemia and hypocalcaemia are uncommon and most infants now bypass the neo-natal intensive care unit. If normo-glycaemia can be maintained throughout the second and third trimesters, present evidence indicates that birth weight and neo-natal metabolic complications are no different from those in healthy women (12).

As peri-natal losses from stillbirths, intra-uterine deaths and respiratory distress syndrome have decreased, so major congenital malformations now account for up to 60% of peri-natal mortality and are between 3 and 5 times as common as in children of non-diabetic women. There is strong evidence that these malformations are the result of hyperglycaemia during the period of organogenesis - between 6 and 12 weeks after conception. I would back this up with two pieces of evidence: (a) the fact that women who have frequent hypoglycaemic reactions (including coma) in the first trimester have a much lower frequency of congenital malformations (13), and (b) the recent experi-ence in East Germany where Fuhrmann and colleagues (14) were able by starting strict diabetic control before conception to achieve a mal-formation rate of only 0.8% compared to 7.5% in women in whom inten-sive care was begun eight weeks or later after conception.

It cannot be stressed too strongly to the woman that the key to preventing peri-natal mortality and congenital abnormalities is to aim for blood glucose concentrations as near to those in the non-diabetic at all times. This inevitably involves an increased risk of hypo-glycaemia which, happily, is not in any way detrimental to the foetus and extremely unlikely to cause permanent injury to the woman her-self.

4.3. Long-term risks to the baby

Prospective parents are likely to be interested in whether their child will eventually develop IDDM and whether, although normal at birth, some subtle damage may appear in future years.

We do not know the exact mechanism of inheritance of IDDM and all we can tell our patients are the empirical risk figures. As far as these go they are relatively reassuring. For example, if a parent has

IDDM, the cumulative risk of IDDM in a child by age 20 to 30 years is somewhere in the range 1 - 6% (15-18). Warram et al. (18) have recently pointed out that several studies, including their own, suggest that IDDM is transmitted less frequently to the offspring of diabetic women than to those of diabetic men. Thus, the cumulative risk of diabetes in the child where the mother is the affected parent is 1.3% compared to 6.1% for the father. The mechanism for this differential inheritance is unknown but possibilities include the lower frequency of recombination between linked loci during gametogenesis in men than in women or alternatively an increased loss of susceptible foetuses in the womb of diabetic women. The risk to full siblings ranges from 3.2 to 5.7% or 10.5 to 12.5% where there is an affected parent in addition to an affected child (17). HLA typing of the whole family would enable the genetic counsellor to refine these risk estimates. Thus, where a sibling is haploidentical with the affected parent or sibling, the risk is very much greater than if the child is HLA non-identical.

There is uncertainty in the literature about whether children of diabetic mothers may later show minor cerebral dysfunction or have a lower IQ. Danish work on children born to insulin-treated diabetic mothers between 1946 and 1966 suggested that the incidence of cerebral palsy and epilepsy might be as much as five times higher than in normal children. An American study (19) of children up to five years of age showed an increased incidence of intellectual delay and concluded that "the presence of acetone in the urine during pregnancy" had a significant, adverse effect on intellectual status. Two studies in the United Kingdom do not support the concept of long-term developmental problems or low IQ in the infants of diabetic mothers (20-21). My conclusion would be that, provided there are no obstetric or neo-natal complications, a diabetic woman should be reassured that the intelligence of her baby is likely to be normal.

4.4. Long term health of the mother

Prospective parents might well decide not to have a family if they knew that, for example, one or other had a high risk of dying or becoming seriously ill within the next 10 years. Where this is likely to be relevant is if the 25 year old woman on whom this section is based has had diabetes since age 2 and has proliferative retinopathy and persistent proteinuria. Such a woman has a high risk of developing end stage renal failure within the next ten years and it is only right that the couple should be appraised of this possibility.

4.5. Cure of diabetes in the mother and its prevention in the child

At present it is not possible to prevent or cure IDDM but the genetic counsellor must give the prospective parents some indication of the likelihood of this happening within the forseeable future. "Cure" of established diabetes by pancreas transplantation is considered elsewhere in this volume. More realistic perhaps is the concept that it might be possible to prevent diabetes in susceptible children by means of immunosuppression (22,23). This would mean identifying susceptible children either by HLA typing or islet cell antibodies (24).

REFERENCES
1. Fraser Roberts JH. An introduction to medical genetics. 6th edition. Blackwells, Oxford, 1973, 269-298.
2. Bengtsson C, Blohme G, Lapidus L et al. Do antihypertensive drugs precipitate diabetes? Brit. Med. J. 1984, 289, 1495-1497.
3. Rimoin DL, and Rotter JL. Genetic syndromes associated with diabetes mellitus and glucose intolerance in "The Genetics of Diabetes Mellitus" ed. Kobberling J and Tattersall R. Academic Press, 1982, 149-181.
4. Tattersall R, Pyke DA and Nerup J. Genetic patterns in diabetes mellitus. Hum. Pathol. 1980, 11, 273-283.
5. Wilson RM, van der Minne P, Deverill I, Heller SR, Gelsthorpe K, Reeves WG and Tattersall RB. Insulin dependence problems in classification in 100 consecutive patients. Diabetic Medicine 1985, in press.
6. Green A and Hougaard P. Epidemiological studies of diabetes mellitus in Denmark: 4 clinical characteristics of insulin-treated diabetes. Diabetologia 1983, 25, 231-234.
7. Heller SR, Lowe JM, Johnson IR, O'Brien PMS, Clarke P, Symonds EM and Tattersall RB. Seven years experience of home management in pregnancy in women with insulin-dependent diabetes. Diabetic Medicine 1984, 1, 199-204.
8. Bromham DR. The increased risk of pre-eclampsia in pregnant diabetics. J. Obstet. Gynecol. 1983, 3, 212-214.
9. Moloney JMB and Drury MI. The effect of pregnancy on the natural course of diabetic retinopathy. Am. J. Opthalmol. 1982, 93, 745.
10. Dibble CM, Kochenour NK, Worley RJ, Tyler FH and Stewart M. Effect of pregnancy on diabetic retinopathy. Obstet. Gynecol. 1984, 59, 699.
11. Prica JH, Hadden DR, Archer DB and Harley JMG. Diabetic retinopathy in pregnancy. Brit. J. Obstet. Gynaecol. 1984, 91, 11.
12. Jovanovic L, Druzin M and Peterson CM. Effect of euglycaemia on the outcome of pregnancy in insulin-dependent women compared with normal control subjects. Am. J. Med. 1981, 71, 921-927.
13. Pedersen J. The pregnant diabetic and her newborn. 2nd edition. Williams & Wilkins, Baltimore.
14. Fuhrmann K, Reiher H, Semmler K, Fischer F, Fischer M and Glockner E. Prevention of congenital malformations in infants of insulin-dependent diabetic mothers. Diabetes Care 1983, 6, 219-223.
15. Degnbol B and Green A. Diabetes mellitus among first and second degree relatives of early onset diabetics. Ann. Hum. Genet. 1978, 42, 25-47.
16. Kobberling J and Bruggeboes B. Prevalence of diabetes among children of insulin-dependent diabetic mothers. Diabetologia 1980, 18, 459-462.
17. Wagener DK, Sacks JM, Laporte RE and MacGregor JM. The Pittsburgh study of insulin-dependent diabetes mellitus: risk for diabetes among relatives of IDDM. Diabetes 1982, 31, 136-144.
18. Warram JH, Krolewski AS, Gottlieb MS and Kahn CR. Differences in risk of IDDM in offspring of diabetic mothers and diabetic fathers. New Eng. J. Med. 1984, 311, 149-152.
19. Stehbens JS, Baker GL and Kitchell M. Outcome at ages 1, 2 and 5 years of children born to diabetic women. Am. J. Obstet. Gynecol. 1977, 127, 408-413.

20. Cummins M and Norrish M. Follow-up of children of diabetic mothers. Arch Dis. Child 1980, 55, 259-264.
21. Hadden DR, Byrne E, Trotter I, Harley JMG, McClure G and McAuley RR. Physical and psychological health of children of type 1 (insulin-dependent) diabetic mothers. Diabetologia 1984, 26, 250-254.
22. Stiller CR, Dupre J, Gent M et al.. Effects of cyclosporine immuno-suppression in insulin-dependent diabetes of recent onset. Science 1984, 223, 1362-1367.
23. Rossini AA. Immunotherapy for insulin-dependent diabetics? New Eng. J. Med. 1983, 308, 333-335.
24. Srikanta S, Ganda OP, Gleason RE, Jackson RA, Soeldner JS and Eisenbarth GS. Pre-type 1 diabetes: Linear loss of beta cell response to intravenous glucose. Diabetes 1984, 33, 717-720.

1.2. Type II Diabetes Mellitus

1.2.1. Introduction: Pathogenesis of type II Diabetes Mellitus
H.M.J. Krans

INTRODUCTION
    The main theme of the next chapters is pathogenesis of type II diabetes mellitus. Insulin secretion, circulating antibodies, effects of other hormones, receptor and postreceptor changes and the role of the nervous system will be discussed. These features are not exclusively related to type II diabetes. The chapters also contain information which is important for the understanding of type I diabetes.
    The distinction between type I and type II diabetes mellitus is primarily made for epidemiological reasons (1). The cause of diabetes mellitus is still not known. In type I the islet of Langerhans is defective. Type II is characterized by a defect in tissue sensitivity and in insulin secretion. It may very well be a conglomerate of various causes and types which have identical clinical symptoms (2).
    Type II diabetes mellitus develops slowly. In the early phase of the disease an occasional increased blood glucose and positive reduction in the urine are found. If during this period insulin levels in the blood are determined, they may be elevated. However, when the insulin level is related to the blood glucose level, insulin sensitivity appears to be decreased (3). Many patients with type II diabetes mellitus have an increased body weight. This complicates investigations on the pathogenesis of diabetes mellitus. The most important data have to be collected from patients who have type II diabetes mellitus without increased body weight (4).

Insulin resistance
    For many years most attention was given to the increased resistance to insulin. More insulin was needed to transport the glucose into the tissues. One of the first hypotheses to explain this phenomenon has been formulated by Randle; the fatty acid cycle (5). The predominant metabolism of fat and fatty acids in the cell and the increased levels of free fatty acids in the blood decrease the uptake of glucose and the effect of insulin on the uptake of glucose. This contributes to the decreased effectivity of insulin and to the development of diabetes in obese patients. The extra amount of insulin necessary to transport sufficient glucose into the cell has to be produced in the islets of Langerhans. The extra continuous strain on the islets could lead to impairment of the synthesis of insulin in the islets and type II diabetes mellitus will develop gradually. But most endocrine organs will hypertrofy and may eventually become autonomous when excessive demands have to be met. If the excessive strain on the islets was the main factor in causing insulin deficiency, diabetes mellitus type II should be seen in all states with increased insulin resistance like : obesity,

Cushing's disease, pregnancy etc. However diabetes mellitus type II does not develop in all patients with obesity or one of the diseases mentioned before. Diabetes mellitus type II has a strong familial appearance. An intrinsic factor in the islets must contribute to the deficient function. A genetic proposition towards diabetes mellitus type II plays an important role (6).

Insulin secretion

The relation between glucose and insulin levels in the blood in type II diabetes is complex. Insulin and glucose values after oral GTT and intravenous GTT, were studied in persons with impaired glucose tolerance tests and normal body weight (4). Persons with obesity were excluded. Consecutive groups of a) controls, b) persons with a borderline abnormal GTT and a normal intravenous GTT, c) with a decreased oral GTT and a normal intravenous GTT, d) with decreased oral and intravenous GTT and e) with type II diabetes were formed. When the consecutive groups were compared the rise in blood glucose was first parallelled by a rise in insulin levels. In the groups with more abnormal GTTs the insulin level was decreased notwithstanding the increased blood glucose. Not all persons with abnormal GTT develop overt diabetes mellitus. Therefore not all persons included in the abnormal groups will become overtly diabetic, but in each group a number of persons will develop diabetes in due time. The islet becomes 'exhausted'.

A change in secretion of insulin can already be demonstrated in a very early phase of the disease and may be pathognomonic. Luft has shown that infusion of glucose induces a two-phasic response of secretion of insulin in normal persons. A rapid phase of increased secretion is seen after a few minutes and a slow phase of increased insulin secretion appears around one hour after glucose injection. In patients who will develop diabetes mellitus type II the first peak has disappeared. This also indicates the change in insulin secretion is a specific phenomenon and not a mere consequence of increased peripheral insulin resistance (7). The regulation of insulin secretion, the relation to metabolic product and insulin resistance is discussed by Pfeiffer.

The secretion of insulin is not a constant process but insulin is secreted in a pulsatile way. The secretion is stimulated (+) or inhibited (-) by various metabolites like glucose (+), fatty acids (+), hormones like glucagon (+), catecholamines through the α-receptors (-) or β-receptors (+), somatostatin (-), or neural messages through the vagus (+) or sympaticus (-) originating from the appetite regulating centres in the brain. The relation between brain and islets is discussed by Steffens.

Receptors

After secretion insulin acts on insulin sensitive tissues like liver, fat, muscle etc. One of the first actions of insulin is binding to specific receptors. The transfer of the insulin message can be inhibited in various ways. Receptor antibodies have been demonstrated as a cause for decreased receptor function, but this is a very rare occurrence (8). These patients show an extreme resistance to exogenous insulin. The specific antibodies may play a role in the origin of diabetes but it is not a common cause.

The response of the tissues on insulin depends on the concentration of insulin that reaches a specific tissue, the number and the affinity of the specific receptors in the tissue. A decrease in receptor number

(9,10) has been described in obese and non-obese type II diabetics. They are most prominent in cells which do not demonstrate a metabolic effect of insulin (monocytes, erythrocytes). In other tissues the reduction of the binding is insufficient to explain the decreased action of insulin. Only ten percent of receptors has to be occupied to express the full action of insulin (11,12). The reduction of binding in tissues like fat tissue etc. is often less than 30%. Moreover in mild diabetes type II no changes in binding are found. Changes in binding are insufficient to explain a presumed insulin resistance in patients with normal body weight. However, when the number of receptors is decreased a higher concentration of insulin is often needed to obtain the same effect; this means a change in sensitivity for insulin.

Postreceptor defects

Another cause of decreased effect of insulin are postreceptor defects (13). This means that the binding of insulin on the receptor has not changed but that somewhere in the chain of intracellular events connected with the binding site one or more steps are decreased in activity. Postreceptor changes affect the translation of the message of insulin into intracellular metabolic changes. A decreased response of insulin in the tissues induces a decreased uptake of glucose in the tissues and an increased bloodglucose level. A postreceptor defect may be caused by a change in the transfer of information from the receptor to intracellular metabolism, through a chain of enzymatic steps, or also by a change of that part of the receptor which is essential for the transfer of the message but does not bind insulin. Often a defect is called a postreceptor defect when changes in cellular metabolism cannot be explained by changes on the binding site. For a further discussion about the role of receptors and postreceptor changes see the chapter written by Wieringa.

Modulation of insulin action

Insulin action may be influenced by various factors as antibodies, hormones etc. Insulin binding antibodies may be induced when exogenous insulin is injected. Spontaneous development of antibodies is not seen as a cause of type II diabetes mellitus. Important hormones which interact with insulin are growth hormone, glucagon, catecholamines, cortisol and some gut hormones. The increased levels of these hormones contribute to the aggravation of the decrease in effectiveness and possibly to the secondary complications of diabetes mellitus. It is debatable if they are the primary cause of type II diabetes mellitus. This is further discussed by Lefebvre.

Some factors which have to be taken into account, but are only marginally treated in the following chapters, are the production of glucose and the islet cell mass. Defective insulin secretion or diminished insulin effectiveness (14,15) may be a cause of diabetes mellitus leading to decreased uptake of glucose into the cells. The level of glucose in the blood is determined by two factors: a) the amount of glucose extracted from the blood into the tissues and b) the amount of glucose entering the blood. The two main sources of blood glucose in the body are the gut (after meals) and the liver. There are indications that in type II diabetes the production of glucose in the liver is increased. Other hormones may also play a role in this process. De Fronzo is one of the investigators who stresses the role of the liver in the metabolic defects of type II diabetes mellitus. This is not further discussed in the following chapters, for the interested reader see references 15 and 16.

In the origin of type I diabetes the main factor is a decrease of the secretion of insulin and this is manifested by degeneration of the B cells in the islets. In type II no changes in the islets can be seen. If peripheral insulin resistance should be the primary cause in diabetes mellitus type II an increase in islet volume should be expected. But in careful studies no hypertrophic islets are found except for some observations in Cushing's disease. The total cellular mass seems to be reduced. Numbers untill 60% are given. This number is sufficient for the production of the necessary insulin, provided that no defect in B-cell function is present (17). It is unclear what the exact defect is. The elevated blood glucose levels may change the capacity of the B-cell to modulate its own secretion (14).

CONCLUSION

We have no answer on the question 'which is the primary defect in diabetes mellitus type II'. Impaired insulin action, changed regulation of B-cell, changes of counterregulatory hormones, in glucose production, in insulin secretion and in cellular mass are all seen. Until now no data are available that indicate which of these factors is the leading factor that induces the changes in the other factors. There is still room for reviews and speculations (2,4,10,15,18).

REFERENCES

1. WHO Expert Committee on Diabetes Mellitus. Second report. Geneva: WHO Tech Rep Ser 646, 1980.

2. Zimmet P: Type 2 (non-insulin-dependent) diabetes - An epidemiological overview. Diabetologia, 22, 1982, 399-411.

3. Kahn CR: Insulin resistance, insulin insensitivity, and insulin unresponsiveness: A necessary distinction. Metabolism, 27 (Suppl. 2), 1978, 1893-1902.

4. Efendíc S, Luft R, Wajngot A: Aspects of the pathogenesis of type 2 diabetes. Endocrine Reviews, 5, 1984, 395-410.

5. Randle PJ, Hales CN, Garland PB, Newsholme EA: The glucose fatty acid cycle. Its role in insulin sensitivity and the metabolic disturbances of diabetes mellitus. The Lancet, ii, 1963, 785-789.

6. Permutt MA, Rotwein P: Analysis of the insulin gene in non-insulin-dependent diabetes. Am. J. Med., November 30th 1983, Proceedings of a symposium, 1-7.

7. Cerasi E, Luft R: 'What is inherited - what is added' hypothesis for the pathogenesis of diabetes mellitus. Diabetes, 16, 1967, 615-627.

8. Kahn CR, Flier JS, Bar RS, Archer JA, Gorden P, Martin MM, Roth J: The syndromes of insulin resistance and acanthosis nigricans. Insulin receptor disorders in man. New Engl. J. Med., 294, 1976, 739-745.

9. Roth J, Kahn CR, Lesniak MA, Gorden P, De Meyts P, Megyesi K, Neville DM, Gavin III JR, Soll AH, Freychet P, Goldfine IE, Bar RS, Archer JA: Receptors for insulin NSILA-s and growth hormone: applications to disease states in man. Rec. Progr. Horm. Res., 31, 1976, 95-126.

10 Kolterman OG, Scarlett JA, Olefsky JM: Insulin resistance in non-insulin-dependent type II diabetes. Clinics in Endocrinology and Metabolism, 11, 1982, 363-388.

11 Kono T, Barham FW: The relationship between insulin-binding capacity of fat cells and the cellular response to insulin: studies with intact and trypsin-treated fat cells. J. Biol. Chem., 246, 1971, 6210-6216.

12 Pedersen O, Gliemann J: Hexose transport in human adipocytes: Factors influencing the response to insulin and kinetics of methyl-glucose and glucose transport. Diabetologia, 20, 1981, 630-635.

13 Bolinder J, Ostman J, Arner P: Postreceptor defects causing insulin resistance in normoinsulinemic non-insulin-dependent diabetes mellitus. Diabetes, 31, 1982, 911-916.

14 Garvey WT, Revers RS, Kolterman OG, Rubenstein AH, Olefsky JM: Modulation of insulin secretion by insulin and glucose in type II diabetes mellitus. J. Clin. Endocrinol. Metab., 60, 1985, 559-568.

15 DeFronzo RA, Ferrannini E: The pathogenesis of non-insulin-dependent diabetes. An update. Medicine, 61, 1982, 125-140.

16 DeFronzo RA, Gunnarsson R, Björkman O, Olsson M, Wahren J: Effects of insulin on peripheral and splanchnic glucose metabolism in non-insulin-dependent (Type II) diabetes mellitus. J. Clin. Invest., 76, 1985, 149-155.

17 Weir GC: Non-insulin-dependent diabetes mellitus: interplay between B-cell inadequacy and insulin resistance. Am. J. Med., 73, 1982, 461-464.

18 Feldberg W, Pyke DA, Stubbs WA: On the origin of non-insulin-dependent diabetes. The Lancet, i, 1985, 1263-1264.

1.2.2. Insulin secretion in noninsulin-dependent Diabetes Mellitus

V. Broadstone, W.K. Ward, J.G. Beard, J.D. Best, J.B. Halter, R. Judzewitsch, D. Porte and M.A. Pfeifer

Impaired insulin secretion is characteristic of Diabetes Mellitus and is responsible for many of the metabolic abnormalities associated with this group of diseases. Nevertheless, the relationship of noninsulin dependent diabetes mellitus (NIDDM) to impaired islet function has been questioned ever since it was shown that the absolute levels of plasma insulin were often normal, or even elevated (1). However, within the past ten years it has become clear that insulin secretion is a complex process with many regulatory controls besides glucose (2,3). As these studies have progressed, it is clear that the determination of the adequacy of insulin secretion is difficult, particularly in the presence of insulin resistance. Therefore, despite the presence of normal or even apparently elevated insulin levels, there is evidence that islet B-cell function is impaired, providing an appropriate analysis of insulin secretion is undertaken (4-7). The regulation of insulin secretion in normal individuals will be reviewed first in order to understand the alterations in the carbohydrate homeostasis in NIDDM.

I. NORMAL PHYSIOLOGY:
   The beta cells (B-cells, which synthesizes insulin in man), the alpha cells (A-cells, which synthesizes glucagon), and delta cells (D-cells, which synthesizes somatostatin) form the major part of the islets of Langerhans. The sequence of B-cell insulin secretion has been studied extensively by histological and biochemical techniques. B-cells respond to a secretory stimulus by movement of stored insulin granules toward the cell surface membrane. Fusion of the vesicle containing the insulin granule with the cell plasma membrane (emiocytosis) then occurs, resulting in liberation of performed insulin granules into the portal venous system and subsequent insulinization of the liver (8). The exact sequence of events that occur between the B-cell stimulus and the secretion of insulin is still unknown, although it is clear that the B-cell can recognize many different stimuli (9,10).
   A. Glucose Stimulation:
   In normal man, glucose stimulation of the B-cell results directly in insulin secretion. A multiphasic islet response to glucose has been demonstrated both in vivo and in vitro (11,12,3). In the classic intravenous glucose tolerance test, the first phase begins after a lag of approximately two minutes and is generally completed by ten minutes. This is called the acute response or first phase response, and is followed by persistent insulin secretion which is called the second phase. Although the second phase of insulin secretion presumably begins at the time of challenge, it is usually not evident until after the first phase has disappeared and is, therefore, usually estimated as the increase in insulin output between 10 minutes and the end of the glucose tolerance test (between 60 and 120 minutes after intravenous glucose administration: Fig. 1). The acute insulin response to

40

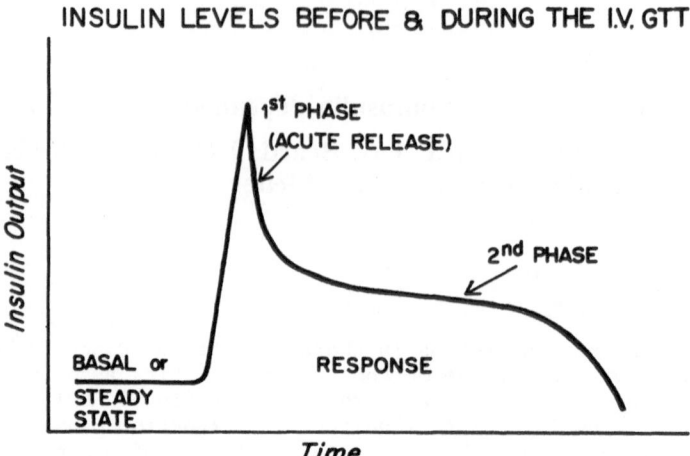

INSULIN LEVELS BEFORE & DURING THE I.V. GTT

Fig. 1

THE BIPHASIC INSULIN RESPONSE TO A CONSTANT GLUCOSE STIMULUS. A theoretical
response to a square wave (constant) change in glucose level is shown. The
peak of the first phase in man is between 3 and 5 minutes and lasts 10
minutes. The second phase begins at 2 minutes but is not evident until 10
minutes has passed. It continues to increase slowly for at least 60 minutes
or until the stimulus stops (3).

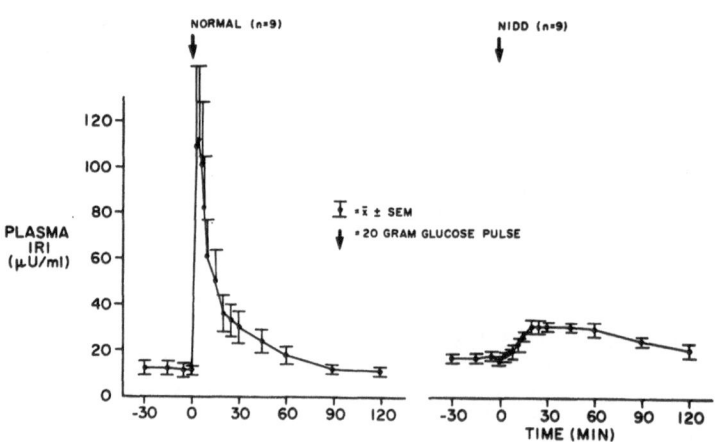

Fig. 2

INSULIN LEVELS DURING 20 GRAM INTRAVENOUS GLUCOSE TOLERANCE TESTS (IVGTT)
IN NORMAL AND NONINSULIN DEPENDENT DIABETICS (NIDD). Fasting plasma glucose
= 85 ± 10 mg/dl in normals and 170 ± 8 mg/dl in NIDD. The first phase is
completely lacking in all NIDDM. The second phase is variably preserved (5).

glucose is directly related to the rate and amount of glucose administration (13). It was originally thought that the first phase represented the secretion of preformed insulin granules and the second the secretion of newly formed insulin. It is now clear, however, that this concept is too simplistic, since in vitro observations suggest that the second phase is the secretion of a combination of preformed and newly synthesized insulin (13,14). The longer the duration of the stimulus, the greater the dependence upon new insulin synthesis. During an intravenous glucose tolerance test, plasma glucose levels are not maintained at a steady elevated level, but decline over time as the additional glucose is cleared from the circulation. This fall of glucose level has no significant effect on the first phase insulin secretion, but reduces the second phase insulin secretion over time until plasma glucose and insulin levels return to their original basal state. Figure 2 demonstrates typical responses from a small group of healthy normal subjects. Note the sharp increase in insulin response during the first phase peaking between three and five minutes and the persistent increase of insulin secretion between 10 and 120 minutes.

If glucose is infused to elevate steady state plasma glucose and insulin secretion rates and a subsequent intravenous glucose tolerance test performed, there is no influence of the prestimulus glucose level on first phase insulin secretion; but second phase insulin secretion is elevated in proportion to the degree of hyperglycemia. Thus, the higher the prestimulus glucose concentration, the greater the glucose levels during the test and the larger the second phase insulin response; and the lower the prestimulus glucose concentration, the lower the glucose levels and the smaller the second phase insulin response. This critical difference between the dependence of first and second phase glucose-induced insulin secretion on pre-stimulus glucose levels in normal subjects is important to understand the abnormality observed in noninsulin dependent diabetes mellitus (5).

When compared with equal amounts of intravenously administered glucose, orally administered glucose causes a greater rise in insulin output (15), an effect likely caused in part by the release of gastrointestinal peptides induced by oral glucose. Gastrointestinal polypeptide (GIP) for example, augments the effect of hyperglycemia to stimulate insulin release, although in the absence of concomitant hyperglycemia, GIP does not cause insulin release (16).   Other gut peptides and neural effects of oral carbohydrate, such as the vagal response to feeding (17), are probably important in enhancing insulin secretion after oral glucose. For several reasons, oral glucose tolerance testing is an inexact method of quantifying pancreatic insulin secretion. First, insulin responses to oral glucose are influenced by gut factors and neural responses to nutrient ingestion, which may vary in magnitude among individuals. Second, gastric emptying and gastrointestinal motility, which also vary among individuals, influence the rate of rise of plasma glucose level and, thus, the rate of B-cell stimulation. Third, the continuous change and variable rise in plasma glucose levels after an oral glucose load make it difficult to compare insulin secretion among different subjects. For these reasons, the oral glucose tolerance test is not the most precise method to quantify B-cell function.

B. NONGLUCOSE REGULATION OF INSULIN SECRETION

1. Glucose as a potentiator of nonglucose stimuli:

Nonglucose stimuli include other nutrient substrates, hormones, and neural regulators. Other nutrient substrates including proteins and their breakdown products (i.e., amino acids), and lipids and their breakdown products (i.e., fatty acids and glycerol) are also direct stimulants of the

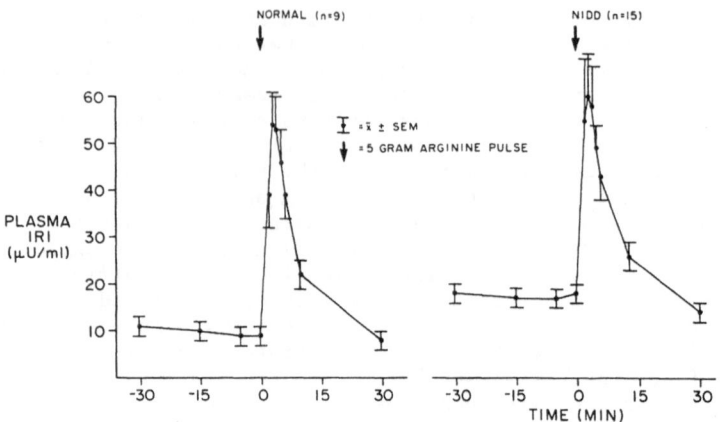

Fig. 3
INSULIN LEVELS BEFORE AND AFTER A 5 GRAM RAPID INJECTION OF ARGININE IN
NORMAL AND NIDDM SUBJECTS. The basal insulin levels of the NIDDM are higher
in proportion to the degree of obesity. NIDDM subjects all had a fasting
plasma glucose less than 250 mg/dl (mean 172 ± 9 mg/dl). The insulin
responses are not different in the two groups (5).

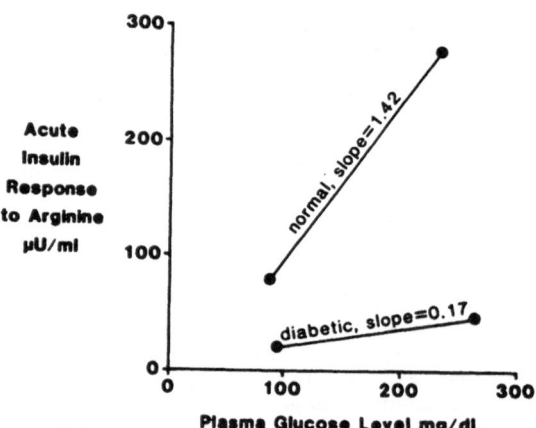

Fig. 4
THE ACUTE INSULIN RESPONSE TO 5 g I.V. ARGININE (MEAN 3-5) MIN INSULIN
INCREMENT) AT TWO PLASMA GLUCOSE LEVELS IN A NORMAL SUBJECT AND IN A WEIGHT
AND AGE MATCHED PATIENT WITH NIDDM. Note that hyperglycemia potentiates
the insulin response to arginine to a greater degree in the normal subject
(Δ acute insulin response ÷ Δ plasma glucose level) is reduced in the
diabetic subject (49).

B-cell. These substances can either be absorbed from the gut or may be endogenously produced. Of the lipids, only free fatty acids and ketone bodies are insulinogenic; and in humans this activity is weak (18). Glycerol is relatively quickly converted to glucose; and this, in turn, results in insulin secretion. Amino acids are far more potent and more important in the response of the B-cell to food ingestion. Most amino acids have been shown to stimulate insulin release. Arginine appears to be the most potent (19) and is commonly used experimentally. An example of the normal insulin response to an intravenous pulse of arginine is shown in the left panel of Figure 3. The response is characterized by an immediate release of insulin which persists for a relatively short period of time (2-10 minutes after injection). The magnitude of this response is critically dependent upon the prestimulus glucose, which will either amplify or suppress this response just as the prestimulus glucose level modulates the second phase of glucose-induced insulin secretion. Thus, despite its similarity in timing to first phase insulin secretion to glucose, it responds metabolically like second phase glucose induced insulin secretion. This dependence of a B-cell response upon plasma glucose level has been called "glucose potentiation" (4).

The magnitude of the acute insulin response to nonglucose stimuli is a nearly linear function of plasma glucose level over the glucose range of approximately 80-300 mg/dl. Accordingly, the slope of the line relating the accute insulin response to a nonglucose stimulus (ordinate) to plasma glucose level (abscissa) can be employed as an index of B-cell responsiveness to glucose (20) (Figure 4). Results have shown that maximal hyperglycemic potention of insulin responses to nonglucose stimuli occurs at a plasma glucose level of approximately 450 mg/dl, since raising plasma glucose above this level causes no further elevation of the acute insulin response to arginine (21). Thus, an acute insulin response to a nonglucose stimulus obtained at a plasma glucose greater than 450 mg/dl is maximal in that it represents maximal potentiation by glucose. This maximal acute insulin response then can serve as an estimate of glucose-regulated B-cell secretory capacity.

2. B-cell as an Integrator:

On the basis of the preceding considerations, one is led to the concept that in man the B-cell works as a metabolic integrator. It integrates food-related nutrient concentrations with neural and hormonal signals to regulate the secretion of insulin and glucagon and ultimately plasma glucose level. The overall islet response is appropriate to the nutrients available, and the environmental circumstances and history of the animal at the time. Thus, even during stress, meals can be eaten and plasma glucose regulated, though at a higher level.

The glucose induced response modification indicates the importance of the regulation of islet cell function by glucose, since prestimulus glucose levels modulates every other secretagogue response. This type of regulation provides for synergism between amino acids and glucose so that when these substrates are ingested together they pass through the portal system to the liver simultaneously with sufficient insulin so that rapid nutrient storage and synthesis can occur.

In addition to glucose and amino acids, many other signals, such as gut hormones, stress hormones, nutrients, and neural factors effect insulin secretion by the B-cell. Insulin itself may have an inhibitory feedback effect on B-cell insulin secretion (22,23), although such an effect has not been demonstrated in all studies (24). It is thought that a major role for the peptide gut hormones is to anticipate nutrient ingestion and

44

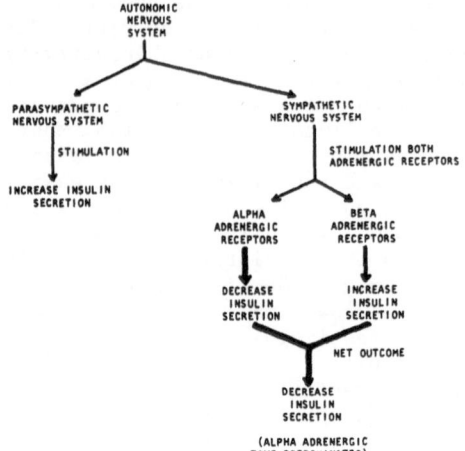

Fig. 5
AUTONOMIC NEURAL CONTROL OF THE PANCREATIC ISLET.

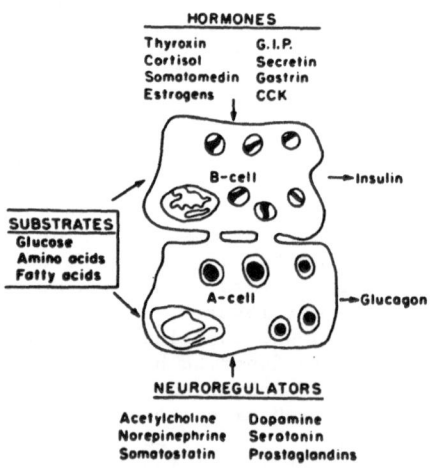

Fig. 6
THE ISLET AS A METABOLIC INTEGRATOR. Substrates such as glucose, amino acids and fatty acids change during meal feeding. The response of the islet to these nutrients (predominantly the former two) is modulated by neural and hormonal signals related to other environmental and/or internal events. The output of glucagon and insulin then regulates the disposition of the nutrients and maintains a regulated plasma glucose concentration at the basal level(26).

stimulate islet function in proportion to their concentration as modulated by the simultaneous concentration of glucose. Thus, hormones such as secretin, gastrin, gastric inhibitory polypeptide and cholycystokinin have all been shown to have insulin stimulatory properties (25) which are sensitive to the circulating concentration of ambient glucose. This glucose potentiation of non-glucose stimulants allows for greater effectiveness of these hormones during periods of nutrient ingestion and reduced effectiveness between meals.

The pancreatic islet is also under autonomic neural control. A schematic illustration is seen in Figure 5. Neuropeptides and acetylcholine released from vagal stimulation are stimulatory to the islet B-cell and are released during nutrient ingestion. They have been shown to be part of a meal anticipatory system related to the sight, smell, and taste of nutrients and provide for islet secretory responses which are greater than the nutrients themselves would stimulate (26). This then tends to minimize the disequilibrium induced by the meal, and minimizes the hyperglycemia and hyperaminoacidemia, which necessarily follow meals.

Although sympathetic stimulation can also cause an increase in insulin secretion by a beta-receptor mechanism (27), alpha -receptor activation inhibits insulin secretion (28). In the pancreatic islet, alpha adrenergic receptor activity predominates over beta-receptor action (29). Thus, during sympathetic activation, insulin release is suppressed, and this is an important factor in the hyperglycemia seen during stress. This adrenergic suppression of insulin secretion during stress can occur both through the sympathetic nerves to the B-cell and local norepinephrine release, and through systemic epinephrine release from the adrenal gland.

Some of the neural regulation of the B-cell is indirect, since both the A-cells producing glucagon and the D-cells producing somatostatin are also under the influence of the autonomic nervous system (30). Pancreatic glucagon secreted from the A-cells has been demonstrated to have insulin stimulatory properties while somatostatin secreted from the D-cells has an inhibitory effect on insulin and glucagon secretion. It has been proposed that alpha adrenergic sympathetic stimulation, while directly suppressing insulin secretion, may also increase islet prostaglandin E which in turn increases islet serotonin which further impairs insulin secretion from the B-cell (31). Figure 6 summarizes all these interactions. The substrates (glucose, amino acids, and fatty acids) are shown as the primary food related nutrient controllers of the islet, with glucose playing a key role since it modulates the sensitivity to the others. These in turn are modulated by all of the hormones and the neural factors relating to the autonomic nervous system including the newly described neuropeptides. These neurohormonal influences are related to the previous history of the animal and its environmental circumstances at the time of nutrient ingestion, as well as to the nutrient ingestion itself. Thus, through regulation of the neuroendocrine system environment influences islet function.

3. Feedback Model for Carbohydrate Metabolism:

In a nonstressed normal subject, who is not taking pharmacologic agents, the basal glucose level will tend to remain the same day after day because of the intrinsic feedback loop shown in Figure 7. For example, any tendency for the glucose concentration to increase is counterbalanced by an increase in insulin secretion and a suppression of glucagon secretion, which regulate hepatic glucose production and tissue glucose uptake to keep the plasma glucose concentration constant. In this way, the insulin and glucose levels are modulated so as to minimize changes in these concentrations while relatively normal production and utilization of glucose are being maintained.

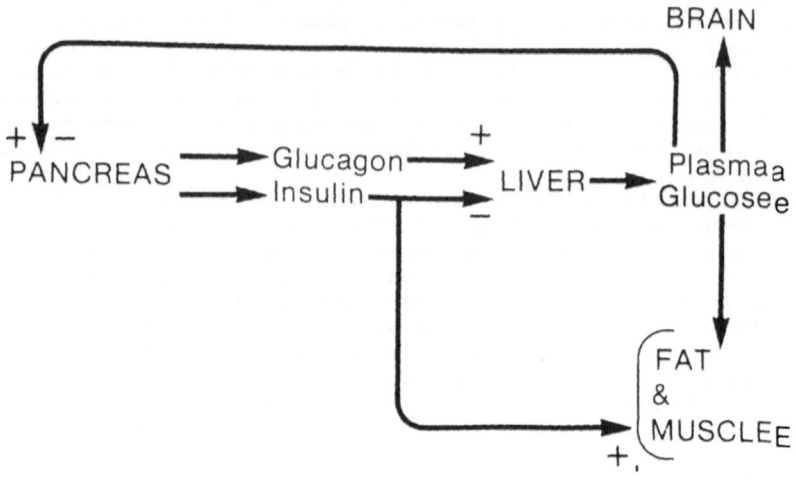

Fig. 7

A FEEDBACK MODEL FOR STEADY STATE REGULATION OF PLASMA GLUCOSE. Glucose
regulates the endocrine pancreas, and in turn, the pancreas regulates hepatic glucose production and peripheral glucose utilization. All other influences on plasma glucose regulation are modified by the operation of this
feedback system (23).

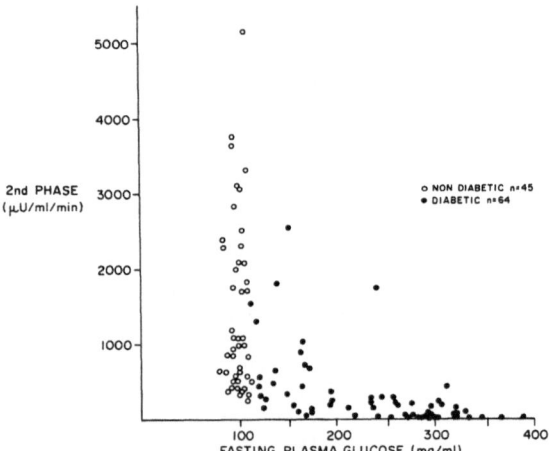

Fig. 8

RELATION BETWEEN FASTING PLASMA GLUCOSE CONCENTRATION AND SECOND PHASE
INSULIN RESPONSES TO A 20 g INTRAVENOUS GLUCOSE TOLERANCE TEST. Similarly
to the nonglucose stimulants, noninsulin-dependent diabetic subjects with
fasting plasma glucose concentrations less than 200 mg/dl (compensated)
tended to have normal responses and those with fasting plasma glucose
concentrations greater than 300 mg/dl (decompensated) had low responses (5).

II. Insulin Secretion in Noninsulin-Dependent Diabetics:

Basal insulin levels in patients with NIDDM as compared with normogly-cemic subjects have usually been reported as normal (33), although elevated (1) and diminished (34) levels have also been reported. However, such comparisons are not entirely straightforward. To accurately compare basal insulin levels in patients with NIDDM with those of normal subjects, the plasma glucose concentration must also be taken into account. Such comparisons have been made in two ways. When normal subjects have been infused with glucose to match their glucose levels and those of diabetic subjects, their resulting steady-state insulin levels have been found to be considerably higher (20). Similarly, when diabetic individuals have received insulin infusions (followed by an insulin washout period) to achieve normo-glycemia, steady-state insulin levels have been found to be lower than those of weight-matched controls (35). Such glycemia-matched comparisons appear to unmask a deficiency of basal insulin output in patients with NIDDM.

Consistent with their generalized subnormal responsiveness to glucose, patients with NIDDM undergo subnormal increments in acute insulin responses to nonglucose stimuli when the plasma glucose level is raised. Thus, as a group, their slopes of glucose potentiation (change in acute insulin response to a nonglucose stimulus per unit change in plasma glucose level) are low (20) (Figure 4). Hence, it appears that a fundamental decrease of basal insulin output exists in NIDDM, but that the resultant hyperglycemia compensates by stimulating basal insulin secretion to a point where insulin levels appear to be normal.

Pancreatic islet function in NIDDM is characterized by decreased responsiveness to a glucose challenge. First-phase insulin release to intravenous glucose is virtually absent in NIDDM (as shown in the right-hand panel of Figure 2) and, in fact, an early absolute decrease in insulin below the basal level is sometimes observed after administration of a glucose pulse. However, second phase insulin secretion is partly preserved; this preservation being dependent on plasma glucose level. As seen in Figure 8, most patients with fasting plasma glucose concentrations less than than 200 mg/dl have a second-phase response to a 20g intravenous glucose tolerance test within the normal range. However, among subjects with fasting plasma glucose concentrations greater then 300 mg/dl, only one patient is within the normal range. Some subjects with fasting plasma glucose concentrations between 200 and 300 mg/dl appear compensated (normal responses) and others are not (low responses).

A. Compensated Noninsulin-Dependent Diabetes (fasting plasma glucose 115 to 200 mg/dl):

When compared to weight-matched euglycemic subjects, these patients usually have normal or nearly normal basal insulin levels. Subjects with fasting plasma glucose concentrations less than 200 mg/dl have nearly normal insulin responses to nonglucose stimuli and second-phase insulin secretion to glucose (Figures 2 & 3). Maintenance of these basal insulin levels and responses is dependent on the potentiating effects of the increased plasma glucose concentrations (Figure 9). Most likely there is an initial decrease in insulin secretion in these patients which results in impaired carbohydrate utilization and increased glucose output by the liver. This, in turn, leads to higher plasma glucose concentrations. The increased plasma glucose compensates for the impairment of islet function by augmenting the insulin response to nonglucose signals and the second phase response to glucose, resulting in an increase to nearly normal insulin responses and maintenance of basal insulin secretion. Providing the defect is not too

48

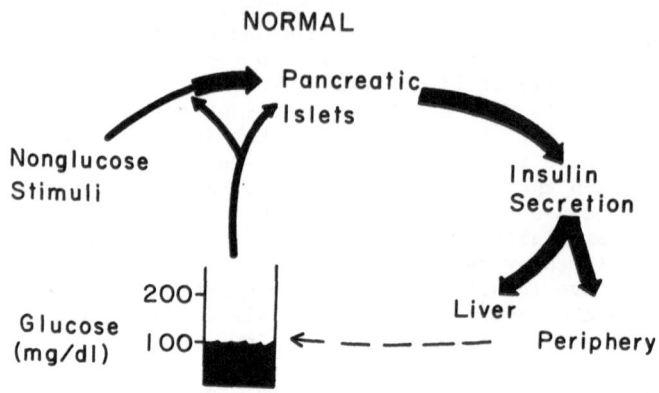

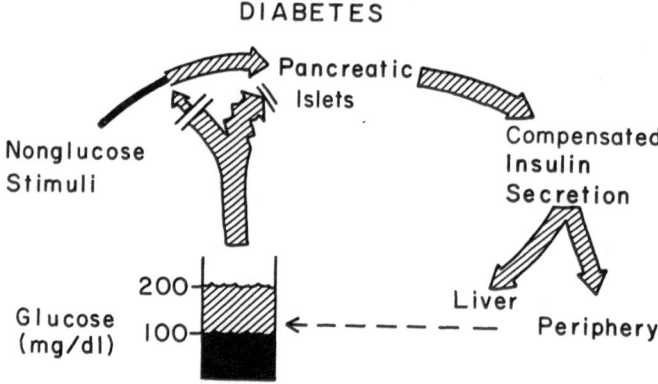

Fig. 9

A SIMPLIFIED MODEL OF INSULIN SECRETION IN NORMAL AND COMPENSATED NONINSULIN
DEPENDENT DIABETICS. Plasma glucose regulated by insulin action in the liver
and periphery feeds back to regulate insulin secretion and impairs glucose
potentiation. As a result of decreased insulin secretion, glucose rises.
This rise compensates for the potentiation defect, but first phase remains
abnormal. Insulin secretion in the basal state and after non-glucose stimulants is compensated, but only at the expense of persistent hyperglycemia.
The height of the fasting plasma glucose is an index of the severity of
the islet lesion. A small deficiency of insulin secretion must still be
present in the basal state, but often cannot be detected (32).

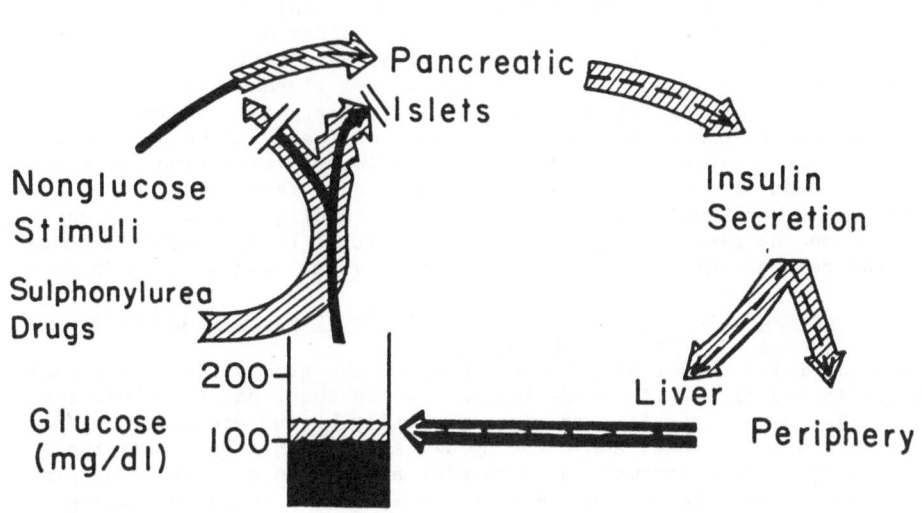

Fig. 10
A MODEL FOR THE ISLET EFFECTS OF SULFONYLUREA DRUGS. Using the feedback
model described in Figure 9, the effect of sulfonylurea drugs is hypothe-
sized to cause an initial increase in insulin secretion which is modulated
as plasma glucose declines. At the new steady state, sensitivity of the
islet to glucose remains increased, but insulin secretion returns to its
original rate, being sustained by the sulfonylurea despite a much lower
glucose level(50).

severe, there is a re-regulated steady state. The feedback between the liver and peripheral tissues remains a closed loop. As a result, carbohydrate production and utilization are restored to normal, but at the expense of the hyperglycemia. During meals, the higher basal glucose level also allows relatively normal responses to nonglucose meal-related stimulants and minimizes the impaired insulin response to a meal. Because of this feedback loop, the fasting plasma glucose concentration is the same day after day in these patients, just as in normal persons (34). There is simply a new higher balance point for the plasma glucose level. The feedback model of islet regulation predicts that the greater the islet defect in an individual, the higher the plasma glucose that will be necessary to maintain a compensated state and near-normal insulin secretion. By this analysis, NIDDM is characterized by a steady-state re-regulation of plasma glucose at higher levels. Because first-phase insulin secretion is not dependent on the glucose level, it is not restored by the higher glucose level and remains the characteristic abnormal islet cell finding in such patients.

B. Decompensated Noninsulin Dependent Diabetes (fasting plasma glucose greater than 300 mg/dl):

When the islet defect becomes very severe, the glucose level necessary to maintain normal insulin secretion may exceed the renal threshold for glucose. The renal excretion of glucose usually begins around 200 mg/dl and is markedly increased above 250 mg/dl. As the contribution of renal excretion of glucose becomes an increasing proportion of total body glucose disposal, the plasma glucose level will reflect to an increasing extent the state of renal function rather than the amount of insulin that is available. Therefore, the low insulin responses observed in diabetics with fasting plasma glucose greater than 300 mg/dl must be due to the renal excretion of glucose and inadequate hyperglycemia to compensate for the islet deficit. Individuals with FPG between 200-300 mg/dl may either be compensated with normal insulin responses or decompensated with deficient responses dependent on the degree of islet impairment and the efficiency of glucose excretion. This would explain the more normal second phase insulin secretion in diabetics with lower fasting plasma glucose and the clear deficiency in those with fasting plasma glucose levels greater the 300 mg/dl. Similar logic would explain the tendency for very hyperglycemic noninsulin dependent diabetics to have low basal insulin secretion for their body weight.

As the glucose level required for the islet compensation exceeds the renal threshold, or as the substrate load of a challenge increases plasma glucose levels above the renal threshold, deficient insulin secretion becomes demonstrable. Under these circumstances there is an open loop system which is unable to provide the stimulus required for compensating insulin responses. The liver responds to inadequate insulin by increasing glucose production further, but this is ineffective in view of the renal glucose losses. As a result, both basal and stimulated insulin secretion and its compensation of second phase and nonglucose stimuli is inadequate, and there is an associated increase in gluconeogenesis, an increase in glucose production by the liver, a decrease in peripheral glucose uptake, and eventually, if the defect is severe enough, loss of the regulation of fatty acid mobilization. This phenomenon is observed when fasting plasma glucose levels are above 300 mg/dl, but can be found in some individuals with very impaired islet function and lower fasting plasma glucose levels if renal glucose excretion is efficient (younger patients). This is almost univers-

ally found in insulin dependent diabetes. In this model of the pathophyso-
logy of NIDDM, it becomes clear that there is an overlap between mild insulin dependent diabetes and severe noninsulin dependent diabetes. In fact,
some patients with insulin dependent diabetes have been described in whom
residual insulin secretion is sufficient to prevent ketoacidosis leading
to a syndrome that is very reminiscent of severe noninsulin dependent
diabetes, while some noninsulin dependent diabetics develop ketoacidosis.
Both types of patients require insulin treatment regardless of the
etilogical distinctions.

C. Relation to Insulin Resistance:

Any change in peripheral insulin sensitivity will have a profound influence on glycemic control (Figure 7). Signals will be transmitted to the islet to increase insulin secretion to overcome the resistance. The hyperinsulinemia found in such insulin resistant states as uremia, Cushing's
syndrome, acromegaly, hypercortisolism, and obesity can be explained this
way. The sensitivity of the normal islet is so great that the increase in
plasma glucose is usually rather mild, but the hyperinsulinemia dramatic.
When this sensitivity is low, such as in NIDDM patients, then the error
signal must be much larger to overcome the impairment in islet function.

The degree of hyperglycemia in a patient with NIDDM is determined by an
interaction between that patient's B-cell sensitivity to glucose and
the degree of tissue sensitivity to insulin since impaired B-cell function
and peripheral insulin resistance frequently co-exist in NIDDM. In the
presence of otherwise normal islet function, isolated insulin resistance
does not generally lead to significant hyperglycemia. In support of this
conclusion is the observation that the vast majority of markedly obese
persons are not hyperglycemic. An explanation for this finding is recent
evidence suggesting that the normal pancreatic islet is capable of increasing its sensitivity to glucose when necessary (36). Therefore, it
appears that the islet lesion is the essential hereditary factor which
then makes the patient susceptible to the impact of insulin resistance
(usually induced by obesity). The etiology of this primary islet lesion
remains to be uncovered (37).

D. Improving B-cell Function in NIDDM   (Sulfonylurea Drugs and
   Insulin Secretion):

Acute administration of sulfonylureas clearly stimulates pancreatic insulin secretion in vitro and in Vivo (38). However, insulin levels have
been reported in some studies to be unchanged during chronic administration
of sulfonylureas (39-42); it has been postulated that the insulinotropic
effects of these drugs are transient. Thus, the major cause of the decrease
of fasting plasma glucose during chronic sulfonylurea therapy has been
ascribed to non-pancreatic effects of the drug (43). A recent demonstration
of the importance of plasma glucose level to the analysis of B-cell
function has led one to challenge the concept that unchanged insulin levels
means unchanged islet function (5). In normal subjects the decrease in
plasma glucose concentration accompanying the administration of tolbutamide
can mask the stimulatory effect of the drug (44).

As a result of these findings in acute studies, one can predict that
early on during sulfonylurea treatment, when plasma glucose levels are
still elevated, that sulfonylurea drugs would cause a persistent absolute
increase in insulin secretion. However, as glucose levels fall during treatment, insulin levels also decline until a new steady state of re-regulated
lower plasma glucose levels are achieved. Although stimulated insulin
levels may decline during treatment, islet function as assessed by B-cell
sensitivity to the potentiating effect of glucose would remain increased.
It has been shown that during chronic chlorpropamide therapy individuals
with pretreatment fasting plasma glucose levels greater than 250 mg/dl

have a persistent increase of basal insulin level during chronic chlorpropamide therapy (45). This persistent increase in insulin secretion is consistent with the concept that these individuals are not able to be completely compensated by their hyperglycemia because their islet defect is
too severe. As the islet defect of these patients is improved by sulfonylurea treatment, fasting plasma glucose levels are now generally below 200
mg/dl and are compensated as a result of a persistent absolute increase in
insulin secretion. The improvement in B-cell glucose sensitivity in diabetics who are compensated to begin with (FPG less than 200 mg/dl) may only
be observed if the challenge is given at the same plasma glucose level
before and after treatment. Thus, the B-cell sensitivity to glucose potentiation, that is the increase in non-glucose stimulant response at matched
blucose levels, is markedly improved even after three to six months of
therapy in all patients. In this sense, the sulfonylurea has substituted
for glucose, allowing for a similar level of insulin secretion while
maintaining a stable re-regulated lower plasma glucose level.

Alterations in other factors important to the regulation of basal plasma
glucose levels such as glucagon secretion (46) or a drug-induced change in
the sensitivity of either liver or peripheral tissues to insulin (43) may
also be present. This would explain why in some individuals the re-regulation of insulin secretion occurs with such small changes in plasma insulin
that an error signal cannot be detected.

Insulin adminsitration for a short period of time improves peripheral
insulin sensitivity (45,48). Thus, it is possible that the initial increase
in insulin levels produce a permanent improvement in insulin sensitivity
which persists during the later phase when insulin levels are lowered to
near their original values.

Regardless of any non-islet effects of these drugs, it is clear that
islet B-cell sensitivity to glucose remains improved (Fig. 10).

III. Summary

In summary, the B-cell of the pancreatic islet functions as a metabolic
integrator for nutrients, such as glucose and amino acids, modulated by
neural and hormonal signals. In normal subjects, glucose directly stimulates insulin release and also augments or potentiates the action of
non-glucose secretagogues. In patients with noninsulin dependent diabetes
mellitus, the direct effect of glucose on insulin secretion is greatly
impaired. However, the basal insulin and insulin responses to non-glucose
B-cell stimulants are maintained at "near-normal" levels, but at the expense of hyperglycemia. A feedback model for the regulation of plasma
glucose has been described. This model can account for the usual stability
of plasma glucose in noninsulin dependent diabetes mellitus and the increased sensitivity of these patients to changes in insulin action. It is
concluded that although altered neuroendocrine control hormones are present
and insulin resistance is common, impaired islet B-cell function is an
essential lesion in noninsulin dependent diabetes mellitus (49). Future
studies will be needed in order to determine the biochemical and genetic
nature of the islet B-cell lesion in NIDDM and its underlying etiology.

The model presented in this text has also been used to explain the
long-term effects of sulfonylurea drugs in this syndrome. Initally, there
is an increase in insulin secretion, but as plasma glucose levels fall, the
augmented B-cell function is masked by the decrease in plasma glucose
concentrations. This improvement in B-cell function can be uncovered by
raising plasma glucose levels to their original elevated state and demonstrating markedly improved insulin secretion in the presence of the
sulfonylurea. Thus, although basal insulin levels and insulin responses to

challenge are often unchanged during long-term therapy with sulfonylureas, it is concluded that a persistent improvement in B-cell function is present and responsible for the major glucose lowering effects of these drugs.

REFERENCES

1. Reaven, G.M., Bernstein, E., Davis, B., and Olefsky, J.M.: Non-ketotic diabetes mellitus: Insulin deficiency or insulin resistance? Am. J. Med. 68:80-86, 1976.

2, Gerich, J.E., Charles, M.A., and Grodsky, G.M.: Regulation of pancreotic insulin and glucagon secretion. Annu. Rev. Physiol. 38:353-388, 1976.

3. Porte, D., Jr., and Halter, J.B.: The endocrine pancreas and diabetes mellitus. In: Textbook of Endocrinology, 6th Edition. R.H. Williams (ed.). Philadelphia, W.B. Saunders Co., 1981, pp 716-843.

4. Halter, J.B., Graf, R.J., and Porte, D., Jr.: Potentiation of insulin secretory responses by plasma glucose levels in man: Evidence that hyperglycemia in diabetes compensates for impaired glucose potentiation. J. Clin. Endocrinol. Metab. 48:946-954, 1979.

5. Pfeifer, M.A., Halter, J.B., and Porte, C., Jr.: Insulin secretion in diabetes mellitus. Am. J. Med. 70:579-588, 1981.

6. Perley, M.J., and Kipnis, D.M.: Plasma insulin responses to oral and intravenous gluocose: Studies in normal and diabetic subjects. J.Clin. Invest. 46:1954-1962, 1967.

7. Turner, R.C., Holman, R.R., Matthews, D.R., Hockaday, T.D.R., and Peto, J.: Insulin deficiency and insulin resistance interaction in diabetes: estimation of their relative contribution by feedback analysis from basal plasma insulin and glucose concentrations. Metabolism 28:1086-1096, 1979.

8. Lacy, P: Beta cell secretion-from the standpoint of a pathobiologist. Diabetes 19:895-905, 1970.

9. Floyd, J., Jr., Fajans, S., Conn, J., Knopf, R., Rull, J.: Stimulation of insulin secretion by amino acids. J. Clin. Invest. 45:1487-1502, 1966.

10. Brown, J., Otte, S.: Gastrointestinal hormones and the control of insulin secretion. Diabetes 27:782-787, 1978.

11. Porte, D., Jr., and Pupo, A.A.: Insulin responses to glucose: evidence for a two pool system in man. J. Clin. Invest. 48:2309-2319, 1969.

12. Grodsky, G.M.: A threshold distribution hypothesis for packet storage of insulin and its mathematical modeling. J. Clin. Invest. 51:2047-2057, 1972.

13. Chen, M., and Porte, D., Jr.: The effect of rate and dose of glucose infusion on the acute insulin response in man. J. Clin. Endocrinol. Metab. 42:1168-1175, 1976.

14. Curry, D.L., Bennett, L.L., and Grodsky, G.M.: Dynamics of insulin secretion by the perfused rat pancreas. Endocrinology 83:572-578, 1968.

15. Elrick, H.: Plasma insulin responses to oral and intravenous glucose administration. J. Clin. Endocrinol. 24:1076-1082, 1964.

16. Verdonk, C.A., Rizza, R.A., Nelson, R.L., Go, V.L.W., Gerich, J.E., and Service, F.J.: Interaction of fat-stimulated gastric inhibitory poly-peptide on pancreatic alpha and beta-cell function. J. Clin. Invest. 66:1119-1125, 1980.

17. Kajinuma, H., Kaneto, A., Kuzuya, T., and Nakal, K.: Effects of methacholine on insulin secretion in man. J. Clin. Invest. 28:1384-1388, 1968.

18. Miles, J., Haymond, M., Gerich, J.: Suppression of glucose production and stimulation of insulin secretion by physiological concentrations of ketone bodies in man. J. Clin. Endocrinol. Metab. 52:34-37, 1981.

19. Floyd, J.C., Jr., Fajans, S.S., Conn, J.W., Knopf, F.F., and Rull, J.: Stimulation of insulin secretion by amino acids. J. Clin. Invest. 45:1487-1502, 1966.

20. Halter, J.Bl, Graf, R.J., and Porte, D., Jr: Potentiation of insulin secretory responses by plasma glucose levels in man: evidence that hyperglycemia in diabetes compensates for impaired glucose potentiation J. Clin. Endocrinol. Metab. 48:946-954, 1979.

21. Ward, W.K., Halter, J.B., Bolgiano, D.C., and Porte, D., Jr: Decreased maximal islet responsiveness to glucose in NIDDM: evidence for loss of secretory capacity. Diabetes 32(suppl. 1): 4A, 1983.

22. Liljenquist, J.E., Horwitz, D.L., Jennings, A.S., Chiasson, J.L., Keller, V., and Rubenstein, A.H.: Inhibition of insulin secretion by exogenous insulin in normal man as demonstrated by C-peptide assay. Diabetes 27:563-570, 1978.

23. Iversen, J., and Miles, D.W.: Evidence for a feedback inbition of insulin on insulin secretion in the isolated, perfused canine pancreas. Diabetes 27:563-570, 1978.

24. Kraegen, E.W., Lazarus, L., and Campbel, J.: Failure of insulin infu-sion during euglycemia to influence endogenous basal insulin secretion, Metabolism 32:622-627, 1983.

25. Dupre, J., Curtis, J.D., Unger, R.H., Waddell, R.W., and Beck, J.C.: Effects of secretin, pancreozymin, or gastrin on the response of the endocrine pancreas to administration of glucose or arginine in man. J. Clin. Invest. 48:745-757, 1969.

26. Woods, S.C., Smith, P.H., and Porte, D., Jr.: The role of the nervous system in metabolic regulation and its effects on diabetes and obesity. In: Handbook of Diabetes Mellitus. Brownlee, M., (ed.). New York, Garland Press, 1981, pp. 109-272.

27. Halter, J., and Porte, D., Jr.: Mechanisms of impaired acute insulin release in adult onset diabetes: studies with isoproterenol and secretin. J. Clin. Endocrinol. Metab. 46:952-960, 1978.

56

28. Robertson, R.P., Halter, J.B., and Porte, D., Jr.: A role for alpha-adrenergic receptors in abnormal insulin secretion in diabetes mellitus. J. Clin. Invest. 57:791-795, 1976.

29. Porte, D., Jr., and Robertson, R.P.: Control of insulin secretion by catecholamines, stress, and the sympathetic nervous system. Fed. Proc. 32:1792-1796, 1973.

30. Samols, E., Weir, G.C.: Adrenergic modulation of pancreatic A, B, and D cells, alpha-adrenergic suppression of beta-adrenergic stimulation of somatostatin secretion, alpha-adrenergic stimulation of glucagon secretion in the perfused dog pancreas. J. Clin. Invest. 63:230-238, 1979.

31. Robertson, R.P., and Guest, R.J.: Reversal by methysergide of inhibition of insulin secretion by prostaglandin E in the dog. J. Clin. Invest. 62:1014-1019, 1978.

32. Halter, J.B., and Porte, D., Jr.: Current concepts of insulin secretion in diabetes mellitus. In: Diabetes Mellitus, Vol. V. New York, American Diabetes Association, 1980.

33. Lerner, R.L., and Porte, D., Jr.: Acute and steady-state insulin responses to glucose in nonebese diabetic subjects. J. Clin. Invest. 51:624-631, 1972.

34. Holman, R.R., and Turner, R.C.: Maintenance of basal plasma glucose and insulin concentrations in maturity-onset diabetes. Diabetes 28:227-230, 1979.

35. Turner, R.C., McCarthy, S.T., Holman, R.R., and Harris, E.: Beta-cell function improved by supplementary basal insulin secretion in mild diabetes. Br. Med. J. 1:1252-1254, 1976.

36. Beard, J.C., Best, J.D., Pfeifer, M.A., Halter, J.B., and Porte, D., Jr.: Corticosteroids alter B-cell sensitivity to hyperglycemia in man. Clin. Res. 30:522A, 1982.

37. Robertson, R.P., and Porte, D., Jr.: The glucose receptor: A defective mechanism in diabetes mellitus distinct from the beta adrenergic receptor. J. Clin. Invest. 52:870-884, 1973.

38. Grodsky, G.M., Epstein, G.H., Franska, R., and Karam, J.H.: Pancreatic action of the sulphonylureas. Fed. Proc. 36:2714-2719, 1977.

39. Seltzer, H.S., Allen, E.W., and Brennan, M.T.: Failure of prolonged sulphonylurea administration to enhance insulinogenic response to glycemic stimulus. Diabetes 14:393-395, 1965.

40. Reaven, G.M., and Dray, J.: Effect of chlorpropamide on serum glucose and immunoreactive insulin concentrations in patients with maturity--onsetdiabetes mellitus. Diabetes 16:487-492, 1967.

41. Chu, P.C., Conway, M.J., et al: The pattern of response of plasma insulin and glucose to meals and fasting during chlorpropamide therapy. Ann. Int. Med. 68:757-769, 1968.

42. Barnes, A.J., Garbien, K.J.T., Crowley, M.F., and Bloom, A.: The effect of short and long term chlorpropamide treatment on insulin release and blood glucose. Lancet 2:69-72, 1974.

43. Olefsky, J.M., and Reaven, G.M.: Effects of sulphonylurea therapy on insulin binding to mononucleated leukocytes of diabetic patients. Am. J. Med. 60:89-95, 1976.

44. Pfeifer, M.A., Halter, J.B., Graf, R., and Porte, D., Jr.: Potentiation of insulin secretion to nonglucose stimuli in normal man by tolbutamide. Diabetes 29:335-340, 1980.

45. Judzewitsch, R.G., Pfeifer, M.A., Best, J.D., Halter, J.B., and Porte, D., Jr.: Chronic chlorpropamide therapy of non-insulin dependent diabetes augments basal and stimulated insulin secretion by increasing islet sensitivity to glucose. J. Clin. Endocrinol. Metab. 55:321-328, 1982.

46. Tsalikian, E., Dunphy, T.W., Bohannon, N.V., Lorenzi, M., Gerich, J.E., Forsham, P.H., Kane, J.P., and Karam, J.A.: The effect of oral antidiabetic therapy on insulin and glucagon responses to a meal. Diabetes 26:314-321, 1977.

47. Scarlett, J.A., Kolterman, O., Gray, S., and Olefsky, J.: Insulin treatment reverses the insulin resistance in type II diabetes mellitus. Clin. Res. 29:97A, 1981.

48. Olefsky, J.O., Ciaraldi, T.P., Kolterman, O.G., and Scarlett, J.A.: Mechanisms of insulin resistance in obesity and non-insulin dependent, type II diabetes mellitus: role of receptor and post-receptor defects. In: Insulin Update. Skyler, J.S., (ed.). Princeton, Experta Medica, 41-73, 1982.

49. Ward, W.K., Beard, J.C., Halter, J.B., Pfeifer, M.A., and Porte, D., Jr.: Pathophysiology of insulin secretion in non-insulin-dependent diabetes mellitus. Diabetes Care 7:491-502, 1984.

50. Pfeifer, M.A., Halter, J.B., Judzewitsch, R.G., Beard, J.C., Best, J.D., Ward, W.K., and Porte, D., Jr.: Acute and chronic effects of sulfonylurea drugs on pancreatic islet function in man. Diabetes Care 7:25-34, 1984.

1.2.3. Insulin antagonism

P.J. Lefebvre and A.S. Luyckx

The present review will deal only with the so-called "circulating insulin
antagonists", the other aspects of insulin resistance such as abnormal
B-cell secretory products or insulin target tissue defects being covered
in other chapters. Circulating insulin antagonists are immunological, hormonal or metabolic, they will be successively considered (see Fig. 1).

1. IMMUNOLOGICAL INSULIN ANTAGONISTS
Immunological insulin antagonists are represented by anti-insulin antibodies and anti-insulin receptor antibodies
1.1.Anti-insulin antibodies
Anti-insulin antibodies most usually result from immunization against
injected exogenous insulin. However, recent investigations (1) have demonstrated that low titers of anti-insulin antibodies are frequently found
in the plasma of type-1 diabetic patients at the time of diagnosis (or
even in some elected cases before the clinical diagnosis of diabetes). In
this particular case, anti-insulin auto-antibodies are considered to be
the consequence of the B-cell damage preceding the clinical onset of diabetes ; due to their low titer, it is unlikely that they exert a significant insulin antagonism. Most of the patients treated with insulin develop
circulating insulin antibodies (2). In terms of immunogenicity the insulins rank in the following order : bovine > porcine > human. Until about
10 years ago, most insulins used in therapeutics were rather impure (3)
and these impurities within the mixture undoubtedly increased their immunogenicity. Switching from "conventional" to "highly purified" insulin preparations is associated with a definite lowering of insulin antibodies
titers and a clearcut reduction in insulin requirements (2) : the higher
the titer of insulin antibodies at the time of switching, the greater the
reduction in insulin requirement thus clearly demonstrating the insulin
antagonism exerted by those antibodies (2).
Several studies have clearly shown that the recently available human insulin preparations are less immunogenic than the purified porcine insulin
preparations (4, 5, 6). In clinical practice, insulin resistance associated with high circulating levels of insulin antibodies is now quite rare.
In addition, various studies have indicated that high titers of insulin
antibodies can act as reservoirs for insulin by binding endogenous or exogenous insulin when it enters the plasma and subsequently releasing it when
low levels of free insulin in the plasma are achieved. The clinical consequences of this phenomena is that patients with antibodies can be relatively protected against acute insulin deficiency (7) (the complex insulin-
antibody functioning as a very long-acting insulin preparation) and that
sometimes insulin is released from the complex at a time when it is not
needed and can therefore favor delayed hypoglycemia (8). Recently, several
authors have emphasized the role of insulin autoimmunity as a cause of

spontaneous hypoglycemia (9).

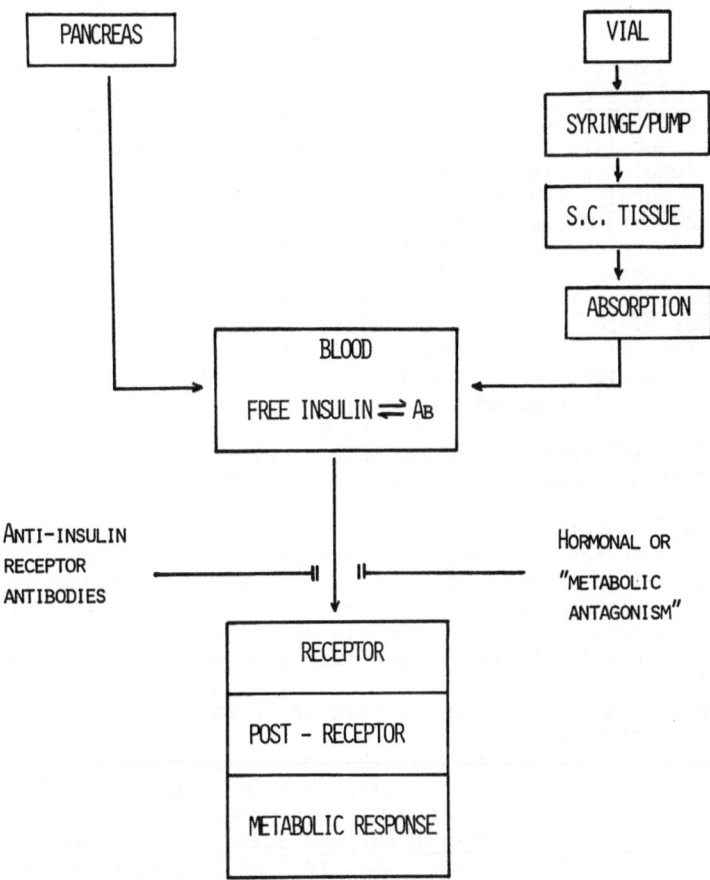

Fig. 1 : Possible sites of insulin antagonism.

1.2.Anti-insulin receptor antibodies

Anti-insulin receptor antibodies were discovered 10 years ago in patients associating severe insulin resistance, hyperinsulinemia, decreased glucose tolerance or frank diabetes and the skin disorders described as "acanthosis nigricans" (10). This rare autoimmune syndrome has been described until now in some 30 patients all over the world.

These autoantibodies to the insulin receptor have greatly helped to our understanding of the receptor structure and function (11).

2.HORMONAL INSULIN ANTAGONISTS

Insulin is quite a unique hormone with its characteristic biological effects which include lowering of blood glucose, stimulation of peripheral

glucose uptake, and inhibition of glycogenolysis, lipolysis and ketogenesis.
Its effects are opposed by the so-called "counterregulatory hormones" cortisol, growth hormone, epinephrine and glucagon which at various levels and
various degrees counteract the action of insulin. Their role can be considered in isolated clinical syndromes of hormonal excess or in the pathophysiology of idiopathic diabetes (review in 12).

2.1.Isolated syndromes of hormonal excess

2.1.1. In Cushing's disease, the glucose intolerance (and in some instances, the diabetes) results from both reduced peripheral glucose clearance and increased liver glucose output. The disease is characterized by
a marked reactional hyperinsulinemia.

2.1.2. In acromegaly, the excess of growth hormone reduces the peripheral
uptake of glucose and increases markedly the liver glucose output, most
of the effects being exerted at the post-receptor level. As in Cushing's
disease, significant hyperinsulinism is a feature of the syndrome.

2.1.3. In pheochromocytoma, the excess of catecholamines (mainly epinephrine) elevates blood glucose by stimulating hepatic glucose output and
inhibiting peripheral glucose uptake (β-effects), an important additional
factor being the inhibition of insulin secretion (mediated through stimulation of α-adrenergic receptors).

2.1.4. In glucagonoma, glucose intolerance or mild diabetes result essentially from increased hepatic glucose output due to inhibition of glycogen
synthesis, and stimulation of glycogenolysis and gluconeogenesis (13).

2.2.In idiopathic diabetes

2.2.1. All counterregulatory hormones are potentially involved in the
pathophysiology of type-1 diabetes. It is now generally recognized that the
high glucagon circulating levels observed in type-1 diabetes are the consequence of the absolute or relative insulin deficiency but that they une-
quivocally contribute to the excessive liver glucose production observed
in diabetes (14).
In addition, glucagon plays a crucial role in orienting the liver metabolic
pathways towards ketogenesis.
Recent studies have demonstrated that the nocturnal surges of growth hormone play a critical role in the relative insulin resistance of the second
half of the night in diabetics, an event usually described as the "Dawn phenomenon" (15). Cortisol and growth hormone seem to be critical in the insulin resistance with hyperglycemia that follows hypoglycemia (Somogyi
phenomenon). An excess of circulating catecholamines is not unusual in
type-1 diabetes, during exercise for instance, and may contribute to the
brittleness of some patients. All counterregulatory hormones are usually
elevated in diabetic ketoacidosis (16).

2.2.2.In type-2 diabetes mellitus, it is classically considered that
"excessive levels of counterregulatory hormones are not an important contri-
butory factor to insulin resistance" (17).

3.METABOLIC INSULIN ANTAGONISTS

More than 20 years ago, Randle *et al*. (18) have provided evidence in
in vitro studies, that high circulating levels of free fatty acids may
impair glucose utilization. This "glucose-fatty acid cycle" concept has
been supported by various studies performed in normal man. Recent investigations performed by Felber and his associates (19) have emphasized the
role that high circulating levels of FFA or high levels of lipid oxidation
may play in the pathogenesis of type-2 diabetes or of the glucose intolerance associated with obesity (Table 1).

TABLE 1. Effect of obesity and diabetes on lipid and glucose oxidation
rates.   Data from Golay *et al.* (19)

	CONTROLS (older group)	OBESE DIABETICS (with excessive insulin response)	OBESE DIABETICS (with defective insulin response)
Total lipid oxidation (G/3h)	4.6 ± 0.6	11.9 ± 1.9	11.2 ± 1.9
	└── 0.001 ──┘		
	└─────── 0.001 ───────┘		
Total glucose oxidation (G/3h)	28 ± 1	31 ± 2	23 ± 2
	└── N.S. ──┘		
	└─────── 0.05 · ───────┘		

During OGTT

4.CONCLUSIONS

The classical insulin antagonists that are the anti-insulin antibodies
and the so-called "counterregulatory hormones" may be involved in the
pathophysiology of some events occuring in type-1 diabetes such as the
transition to diabetic ketoacidosis or the Dawn phenomenon or the Somogyi
phenomenon.   In contrast, their role in the pathophysiology of type-2 diabetes remains entirely hypothetical ; in that form of diabetes, abnormalities seem to occur essentially at the level of the mechanisms controlling
insulin release from the B-cell and/or at the site of action of insulin on
its target tissues.

REFERENCES

1. Palmer JP, Asplin CM, Clemons P, Lyen K, Tatpati O, Raghu P, Paquette
   TL. Insulin antibodies in insulin-dependent diabetics before insulin
   treatment. Science 1983, 222, 1337-1339
2. Luyckx AS, Daubresse JC, Lefèbvre P. L'intérêt des insulines monocompo-
   sées dans le traitement du diabète. Med. Hyg. 1974, 32, 1283-1286
3. Bloom SR, Adrian TE, Mitchell SJ, Barnes AJ, Polak JM. Dirty insulin,
   a stimulant to autoimmunity. Gut 1976, 17, 817
4. Fineberg SE, Galloway JA, Fineberg NS, Rathbun MJ, Hufferd S. Immuno-
   ginecity of recombinant DNA human insulin. Diabetologia 1983, 25, 465-
   469
5. Schernthaner G., Borkenstein M, Schober E, Fink M. Immunogenicity of
   human monocomponent insulin in man : long-term follow-up of 77 newly
   treated type 1 (insulin-dependent) diabetic patients. Diabetologia 1983
   25, 192
6. Luyckx AS, Daubresse JC, Jaminet C, Scheen A, Lefèbvre PJ. Immunogenicity of semisynthetic human insulin in man. Long-term comparison with
   porcine monocomponent insulin. Diab. Metab. (Paris) (submitted)
7. Vaughan NJA, Matthews JA, Kurz AB, Nabarro JDN. The bioavailability of
   circulating antibody-bound insulin following insulin withdrawal in type
   1 (insulin-dependent) diabetes. Diabetologia 1983, 24, 355-358
8. Madsbad et al. Personal communication
9. Benson E.A., Ho P, Wang C, Wu PC, Fredlund PN. Insulin autoimmunity as

a cause of hypoglycemia. Arch. Intern. Med. 1984, 144, 2351-2354
10. Flier JS, Kahn CR, Roth J, Bar RS. Antibodies that impair insulin receptor binding in an unusual diabetic syndrome with severe insulin resistance. Science 1975, 190, 63-65
11. Kasuga M, Karlsson FA, Kahn CR. Insulin stimulates the phosphorylation of the 95,000 dalton subunit of its own receptor. Science 1982, 215, 185-187
12. Schade DS, Eaton RP, Alberti KGMM, Johnston DG. Diabetic coma. University of New Mexico Press, Albuquerque, N.M., U.S.A. 1981, 250 pages.
13. Luyckx AS, Lefèbvre PJ. Les glucagonomes. Diab. Metab. 1981, 7, 289-300
14. Lefèbvre PJ, Luyckx AS. Glucagon and diabetes : a reappraisal. Diabetologia 1979, 16, 347-354
15. Campbell PJ, Bolli GB, Cryer PE, Gerich JE. Nocturnal spikes in growth hormone secretion cause the dawn phenomenon. Diabetologia 1984, 27, 262
16. Schade DS, Eaton RP. Pathogenesis of diabetic ketoacidosis : a reappraisal. Diabetes Care 1979, 2, 296-306
17. Olefsky JM. Insulin antagonists and resistance. In Diabetes Mellitus. Theory and Practice. 3rd Ed. Medic. Examin. Publish. Co., New-York, U.S.A., 1983, 151-178
18. Randle PJ, Hales CN, Garland PB, Newsholme EA. The glucose fatty-acid cycle its role in insulin sensitivity and the metabolic disturbances of diabetes mellitus. Lancet 1963, i, 785-789
19. Golay A, Felber JP, Meyer HU, Curchod B, Maeder E, Jequier E. Study on lipid metabolism in obesity diabetes. Metabolism 1984, 33, 111-116

1.2.4. The contribution of the central nervous system to the regulation of insulin release and the stabilization of blood glucose

A.B. Steffens and P.G.M. Luiten

1. NEUROANATOMY

1.1. Introduction

It has become a widely established notion that the central nervous control of feeding and metabolism is one of the major functions of the limbic system. Profound changes in food- and water-intake, body weight and body composition can be achieved by lesions or stimulations in various limbic structures such as amygdaloid body, prefrontal cortex, septum, limbic midbrain and most significantly in the hypothalamus (1, 4, 10, 11, 19, 23, 24). In summarizing a vast body of evidence, the hypothalamus must be regarded as the major final output structure of the limbic brain by which it influences the autonomic nervous system and the neuroendocrine pathways.

A number of studies now have provided strong evidence that the nervous control of feeding and homeostatic functions is the result of highly sensitive neural control of endocrine mechanisms (27, 34, 35). As most relevant hormonal systems related to feeding, body weight and metabolism we should consider the hormones released from the islets of Langerhans in the pancreas and the hormones of the adrenal glands. Both physiological and anatomical data in recent years point at a close relation between pancreatic endocrine mechanisms and the adrenal endocrine system both in normal and pathological diabetic situations (2, 3, 9, 33).

As part of the present survey on the nervous control of the pancreatic B-cell, we therefore will present here an overall picture of the organization of neural pathways innervating the endocrine pancreas and adrenal glands. At the level of the hypothalamus a distinction can be made between cell groups that provide access to the autonomic nervous system and cell population more directly linked to the neuroendocrine pathway. The ventromedial (VMH), lateral (LHA) and part of the paraventricular nuclei (PVP) can be considered as nuclei related to the sympathetic or parasympathetic autonomic nervous system (11, 12, 35). Parts of the paraventricular nucleus and median eminence on the other hand constitute the major links to the neuroendocrine system (14, 17).

1.2. Procedures

The anatomical pathways originating from the above-mentioned hypothalamic nuclei towards their target structures in pancreas and adrenals have been analyzed by means of a variety of intra-axonal transport techniques. Most of the data presented here are based on retrograde transport (from synapse to cell body) of horseradish peroxidase (HRP) and anterograde transport (from cell body to synapse) of radio labeled aminoacids (^{3}H-Leucine) or Phaseolus vulgaris leuco-agglutinin (PHA-L) (31, 32). The PHA-L method is a recently developed technique based on active uptake by the soma membrane of the lectin PHA-L, then the anterograde labeling by the lectin of axon and terminal synaptic boutons, followed by immunocytochemical vizualization of the labeling. The present data are obtained from approx. 200 experiments all carried out on male albino Wistar rats of 300 gm weight. Following the appropriate survival times that varied between 1 day for the HRP and 14 days for the ^{3}H-Leucine experiments, the brains were fixed by transcardial perfusions of buffered aldehyde mixtures. Frozen sections were treated according to histochemical (HRP), autoradiographic (^{3}H-Leu) or immunocyto-chemical (PHA-L) procedures.

1.3. Nervous innervation

1.3.1. Autonomic innervation of the pancreas, the pancreatic B-cell and the adrenal gland. The preganglionic innervation of pancreas and adrenals were studied after injections in these organs with HRP (15). After application of this tracer to the adrenal gland preganglionic labeling occurred in intermediolateral cell column (IML) of segments of the thoraco-lumbar spinal cord. The labeled cells together constitute a longitudinal column that is strictly ipsilaterally organized. After HRP injections in the adrenal gland we never observed any labeling in parasympathetic nuclei of the brainstem.

The pancreas, on the other hand, was shown to be innervated by both or-tho- and parasympathetic components of the autonomic nervous system. After HRP injections in the pancreas bilateral contingents of labeled sympathetic nerve cells were observed in the intermediolateral and intermedio-medial (area 10 of Rexed) of the segments thoracic 2 - lumbar 3 of the cord. Apart from this sympathetic cell group numerous labeling appeared in the parasym-pathetic ambiguus and dorsal motor vagus nucleus (10 in Fig. 1). To deter-mine the position of preganglionic cells that innervate the pancreatic B-cell we compared the innervation of the normal pancreas with the innerva-tion of the alloxan-diabetic pancreas (15). Treatment with alloxan results in a considerable decrease of cellular labeling in the nucleus ambiguus and in particular in the left dorsal motor vagus nucleus as a result of B-cell destruction and its innervation.

1.3.2. Parasympathetic pathways from hypothalamus to pancreas. After having established the position of parasympathetic neurons in the lower brainstem that innervate the endocrine pancreas, we studied the descending pathways originating from the lateral hypothalamic area (LH), which we con-sidered as the parasympathetic representative in the hypothalamus. Direct axonal connections could be demonstrated between the LH and the motor neur-ons in the ambiguus and dorsal motor vagus nucleus. A more extensive connec-tion, however, is formed by projections from LH with the parvocellular re-ticular formation (RET) of the lower brainstem (31). This reticular forma-tion proved to be a major relay between LH and the parasympathetic motor nuclei.

1.3.3. Sympathetic pathways from hypothalamus to pancreas. The major sym-pathetic outflow pathway of the hypothalamus originates from the ventrome-dial nucleus (VN) that was shown to have a dominant projection to the peri-aqueductal gray in the mesencephalon (PAG) (13). The PAG maintains a dense and circumscript efferent connection to the parvocellular reticular nucleus in the lower medulla oblongata (RET). This reticular nucleus possesses a well-organized variety of outgoing connections. A vast contingent of fibers can be seen leaving the more ventral aspects of the reticular formation to take a descending course in the lateral funiculus of the cord. A rich pattern of labeled terminal fibers and boutons in the intermediolateral column after tracer injections in the parvocellular reticular formation de-monstrates the existence of a sympathetic descending circuit. In summary, this circuit originates in the ventromedial hypothalamus and via the peri-

VMH AND LHA ORIGINATING PATHWAYS

FOR RELEASE OF PANCREATIC HORMONES

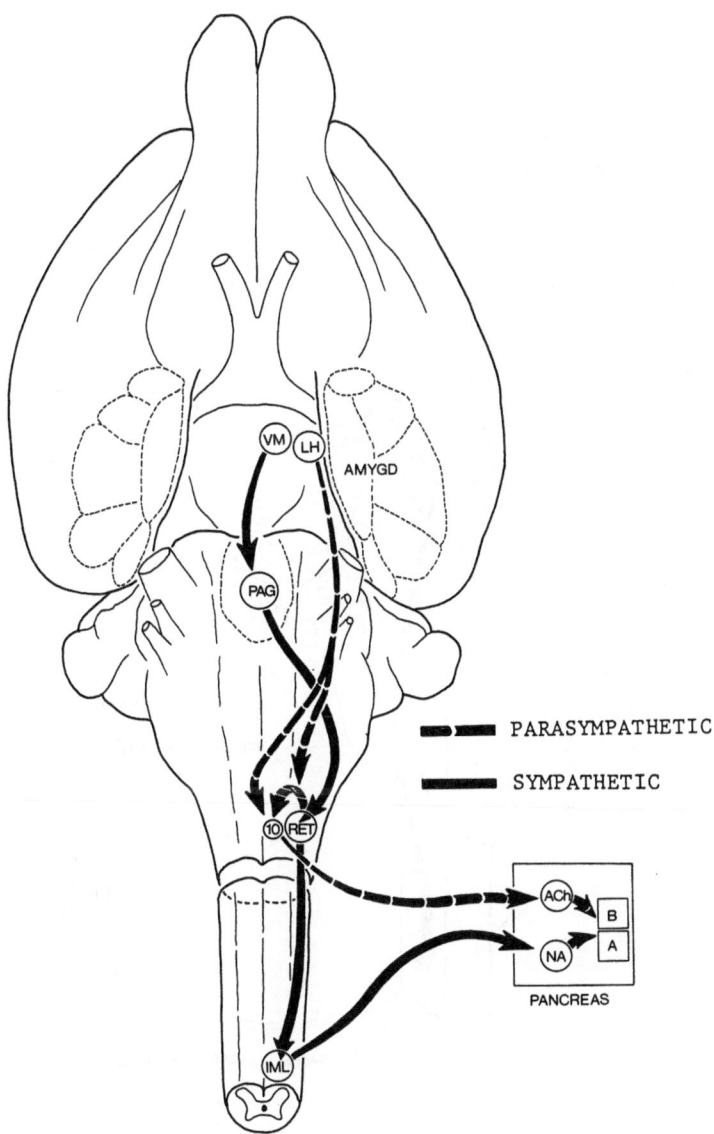

Fig.1. Survey of neural pathways between ventromedial (VM) and lateral hypothalamus (LH) and the endocrine pancreas. Other abbreviations: A - pancreatic A-cell; ACh - cholinergic postganglionic neuron; B - pancreatic B-cell; IML - intermediolateral column; NA - noradrenergic sympathetic postganglionic neuron; PAG - periaqueductal gray; RET - parvocellular reticular formation; 10 - dorsal motor vagus and ambiguus nuclei.

PATHWAYS FOR RELEASE OF ADRENAL HORMONES

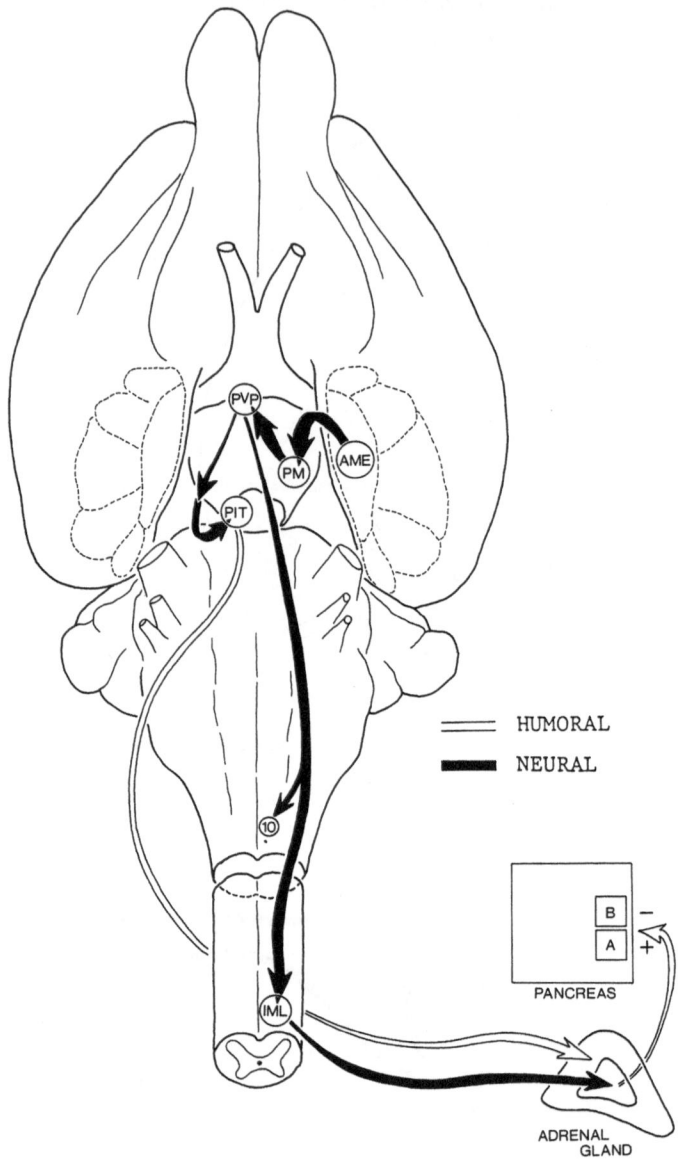

Fig. 2. Survey of pathways for the release of adrenal hormones. Abbreviations: A - pancreatic A-cell; AME - medial amygdala; B - pancreatic B-cell; IML - intermediolateral column; PIT - anterior pituitary; PM - ventral premammillary nucleus; PVP - parvocellular paraventricular nucleus of the hypothalamus; 10 - dorsal motor vagus and ambiguus nucleus.

aqueductal gray reached the medullary reticular formation. The latter
structure forms a final link with the intermediolateral column.

1.3.4. <u>Descending autonomic pathways of the paraventricular hypothalamic
nucleus</u>. Recent investigations of this nucleus have demonstrated
that the PVN is the most powerful site to elicit feeding behavior by chemical stimulation (11). The connections of the PVN show that this nucleus
also is in the unique position both to have direct access to the autonomic
nervous system and to neuroendocrine systems. The pathways that link the
PVN to the autonomic nervous system consist of two fiber systems that without interruption travel through the entire brainstem and spinal cord. At
all autonomic centers on their descending course these fibers terminate
heavily and thus provide the hypothalamus with a direct outflow circuit to
para- and orthosympathetic cell groups (14, 31). It has recently been
shown that the PVN on the parasympathetic neurons in the ambiguus nuclei
exerts an inhibitory influence. Furthermore, it is most likely that the
PVN-sympathetic connection relates the hypothalamus directly not only with
preganglionic cell groups that innervate the endocrine pancreas, but also
with sympathetic preganglionic neurons of the adrenal medulla being responsible for epinephrine release (14).

1.3.5. <u>Neuroendocrine pathways to the adrenal cortex</u>. From physiological
analysis it must be concluded that serum levels of corticosteroids released from the adrenal cortex are of great importance for the release of
pancreatic hormones and metabolism in general and in diabetic cases in particular (2, 33). It is assumed so far that the adrenal cortex does not receive a direct autonomic innervation but is under control of neuroendocrine
pathways. In the neuroendocrine system the paraventricular hypothalamic nucleus plays a key role by its corticotropin-releasing-factor (CRF) containing cell groups. These CRF cells of the PVN project heavily on the vascular
system in the external laminae of the median eminence (17). The CRF that
reach this portal vein system of the pituitary are responsible for the release of adreno corticotropic hormone (ACTH) from the adenohypophysis and
thus stimulate the secretion of corticosteroids. It is worth mentioning here
that it has been shown that secretion of insulin is stimulated by corticotropin releasing factor in experimental rats (33).

2. CNS TRIGGERED INSULIN AND GLUCAGON RELEASE
2.1. <u>Contribution of the autonomic nervous system</u>

As described in previous paragraphs the islet of Langerhans receives an
important innervation by the sympathetic and parasympathetic division of
the autonomic nervous system. A large body of evidence is available at present that the autonomic nervous system controls the hormone output of the
islet of Langerhans apart from the familiar factors as: 1°. a rise of
blood glucose above a basal value of 100 mg/dl, 2°. a rise of some amino-
acids like alanine, arginine, and ornithine provided the presence of a normal basal blood glucose level (18), 3°. release of gut hormones especially
cholecystonikin (CCK), gastrin and gastric inhibitory peptide (GIP) (5).

The first indications of a contribution of the cns were obtained in 1967
by Kaneto et al. (6) who showed that electric stimulation of the vagus
nerve to the islet of Langerhans elicited insulin release. Since that time
it is well established that the islet of Langerhans is under continuous
sympathetic and parasympathetic control. Vagal activity induces insulin release by activation of the B cell, whereas sympathetic activity elicits
glucagon release from the A cell (8) and suppresses insulin release from
the B cell by an α_2 adrenoreceptor mechanism (21). However, evidence is
available that also vagal activation might contribute to glucagon release,

68

at least in dog (7). Apart from the insulin release suppressing effect by activation of α₂ adrenoreceptors on the B cell insulin release can be activated by a β₂ adrenoreceptor mechanism (8, 22). Glucose loads administered during β₂-adrenergic stimulation of the B cell do not elicit glucose-induced insulin release which is apparently inhibited by the α₂-adrenoreceptor stimulating property of the catecholamines. In this respect the sympathetic innervation of the adrenal medulla is most important since its activation triggers release of norepinephrine (NE) and epinephrine (E) into the blood circulation. The adrenal medulla contributes to the control of insulin and glucagon release, not only by immediate effects of NE and E on the α₂ and β₂ adrenoreceptors on A and B cells of the islet of Langerhans but also by the effects of E and NE on the glycogenolysis in the liver which is mediated by a β₂ adrenoreceptor mechanism in rat and results in an increase in blood glucose (28).

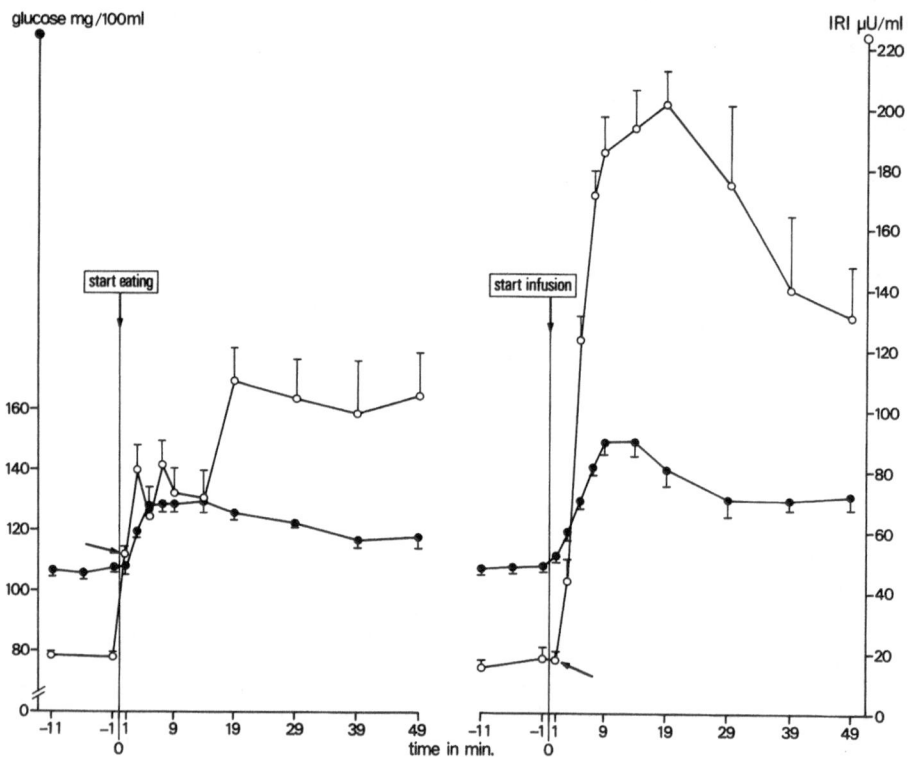

Fig. 3. Left: blood glucose (●) and plasma insulin (o) levels during oral ingestion of carbohydrate rich fluid food. Start of meal at time zero. Right: blood glucose (●) and plasma insulin (o) levels during intragastric infusion of carbohydrate rich fluid food. Entrance of fluid into the stomach at time zero. Arrow indicates insulin level 1 min after start of ingestion or stomach infusion of food (N = 6) (From Steffens, 1976).

2.2. The role of the CNS

Control exerted by activation of the autonomic nervous system on the islet of Langerhans must have its origin in the central nervous system as appears from the following experiments. Food intake elicits an increase in insulin already in the first minute after onset of food intake whereas glucose starts to rise in the third minute (Fig. 3, left panel). The anticipatory early insulin response (EIR) must be attributed to an oropharyngeal reflex in which the cns participates, as appears from the following observations. Rats provided with stomach catheters were habituated to eat a fluid carbohydrate-rich test meal and the quantity eaten and the time required to do so were measured. In the second part of this experiment the same animals received the fluid carbohydrate-rich test food directly in the stomach via a chronic stomach catheter. The same quantity of food as eaten during the oral test meal was infused via the stomach catheter at the same rate needed for oral consumption. When the rats consumed the food, glucose rose in the third minute and an EIR was present, as Fig. 3 shows (26). When the food was infused into the stomach glucose also rose in the third minute and the speed of increase was the same as that for oral consumption. However, in the infusion experiment glucose continued to rise to 150 mg/dl whereas when food was taken orally, glucose levelled off at 130 mg/dl (26). An EIR was present after oral consumption, but was absent when food was infused into the stomach. A second rise in insulin occurred in the oral intake experiment and reached a maximum value of about 100 µU/ml plasma. In the infusion experiment in which an EIR was absent, insulin started to rise in the third minute and followed the increase in glucose levels. It continued to rise to 200 µU/ml plasma.

Similar results were obtained in alloxan diabetic rats recovered from diabetes by fetal pancreas transplants under the kidney capsula (30). As Fig. 4 shows, the recovered rats, as opposed to a group of control rats, did not have an EIR during a meal and the pattern of the insulin and glucose curve during and after a meal was very similar to those of rats that received the food immediately in the stomach (cf. Figs. 3 and 4). These results clearly show that the exaggerated rise in glucose after a meal in rats with pancreas transplants contributes to the exaggerated insulin response.

Evidently when either the afferent pathway (as in the stomach tube fed rats) or the efferent pathways (as in rats with pancreas transplants) of the reflex arc responsible for insulin release is interrupted the insulin and glucose profiles during and after a meal are too large as compared to the situation in normal rats. Presumably lack of an EIR is responsible for this situation.

2.3. The role of the hypothalamus

As relay station in the reflex arc between oral cavity and the islets of Langerhans serve probably several areas of the hypothalamus as appears from the following observations. Axons transmitting gustatory signals reach the pontine taste area in the parabrachial nucleus (PBN) via the nucleus tractus solitarius (NTS) (20). Several hypothalamic areas, the lateral hypothalamic area (LHA), the dorsomedial hypothalamus (DMH) and the nucleus paraventricularis (PVN) receive afferent fibers from the PBN and NTS (20). As described in paragraph 2 of this survey the islet of Langerhans and the adrenal medulla receive many projections of these hypothalamic areas and the ventromedial hypothalamic area (VMH). Moreover, VMH lesion leads to increased activity of the vagal pancreatic nerve and reduced activity of the splanchnic nerve (35). On the other hand, lesion of the LHA results in decreased pancreatic vagal activity, and produces either decreased or in-

70

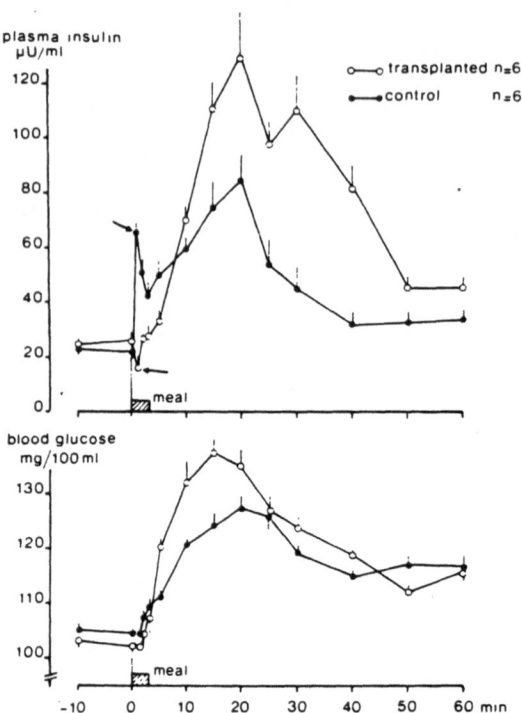

SPONTANEOUS FOOD INTAKE

Fig. 4. Comparison of plasma
insulin and blood glucose
responses between control
(●) and transplanted (o)
rats (N = 6). The figure
shows the effect of food intake in the fed state.
(From Strubbe and van Wachem
1981.)

creased activity of the pancreatic splanchnic nerve (35).

Taking these observations into account it is not surprising that the hypothalamus plays a key role in the nervous control of the islet of Langerhans. Since the hypothalamus contains many noradrenergic neurons and food
intake elicits an immediate release of norepinephrine in several hypothalamic areas (16, 34) it is not surprising to find that infusion of NE into
the LHA in minute quantities results in an immediate rise in plasma insulin (see Fig. 5). This insulin rise is of a parasympathetic origin because
atropinization of the rat before infusion of NE into the LHA suppresses the
insulin response completely (29). Food intake during infusion of NE into
the LHA leads to an exaggerated insulin response (29) (see Fig. 6). Infusion of NE into the VMH on the other hand, leads to an increase in plasma
glucagon (27). It is reasonable to suppose that food intake leads to an immediate rise in NE release in LHA neurons which in its turn increases insulin output from the B cell of the islet of Langerhans, resulting in an EIR.
The EIR probably contributes to the uptake of absorbed glucose from a newly
ingested meal by promotion of glycogenesis in the liver. The increased
liver glycogenesis prevents leakage of glucose into the general circulation
so that 1) the B cell of the islet of Langerhans is not overloaded, 2) the
flow of absorbed glucose during digestion is not directed to the fat re-
serves into a large extent.

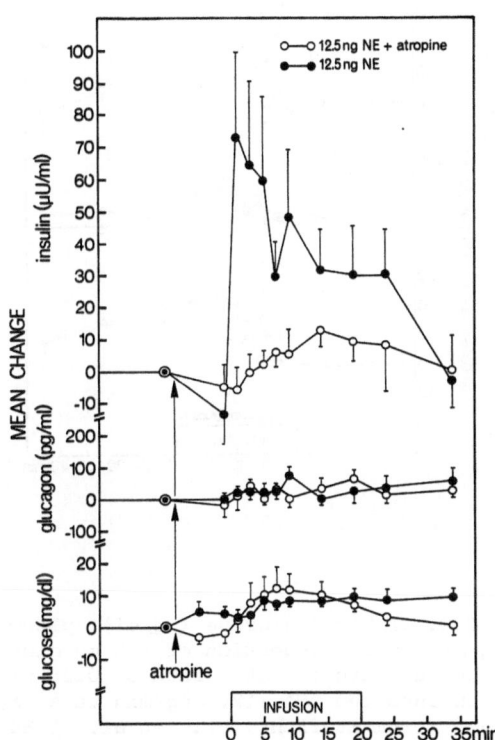

Fig. 5. Effect of NE infusion in the LHA (12.5 ng/min at rate of 0.25 μl/min during 20 min) on blood glucose, plasma insulin and glucagon either with atropinization (0.5 mg/kg), o—o or without atropinization, ●—●. Data are expressed as means ± S.E. mg/dl, μl/ml, pg/ml respectively, changes from pre-atropinization levels of glucose, insulin and glucagon which were the average of these time point 1 min before atropinization. (From Steffens, Flik et al., 1984.)

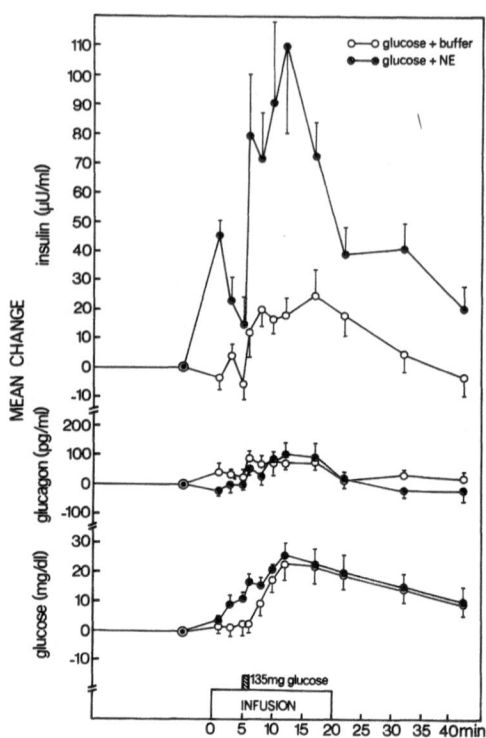

Fig. 6. Mean changes ± S.E. of blood glucose (mg/dl), plasma insulin (μU/ml) and plasma glucagon (pg/ml) during ingestion of 135 mg glucose which was ingested during either buffer infusion at a rate of 0.25 μl/min during 20 min, o—o, or NE infusion into the LHA (12.5 ng/min at a rate of 0.25 μl/min during 20 min), ●—●. (From Steffens, Flik et al., 1984.)

3. CONCLUSIONS

From the preceding paragraphs it is clear that ample evidence is present that the hypothalamus contributes to the control of the islet of Langerhans via parasympathetic and sympathetic pathways. The aim of this control by the autonomic nervous system is probably to achieve an accurate regulation of both the hormone output by the islet of Langerhans and the blood sugar level. Besides its effects on the islet of Langerhans, the autonomic nervous system is also able to affect directly glycogenolysis and glycogenesis in the liver as appears from the work of Shimazu (25) so that the autonomic nervous system may regulate blood glucose levels also directly without interference of hormones from the islet of Langerhans.

REFERENCES

1. Box MB and Mogenson GJ: Alterations of ingestive behaviours after bilateral lesions of the amygdala in the rat. Physiol Behav. 15 (1975) 679-688.
2. Cameron OG, Kronfol Z, Greden JF and Carroll BJ: Hypothalamic-Pituitary-Adrenocortical activity in patients with diabetes mellitus. Arch Gen Psychiatry 41 (1984) 1090-1095.
3. Dallman MF: Viewing the ventromedial hypothalamus from the adrenal gland. Am J Physiol. 246 (1984) R1-R12.
4. Gordon FJ and Johnson AK: Electrical stimulation of the septal area in the rat: prolonged suppression of water-intake and correlation with self-stimulation. Brain Res. 206 (1981) 421-430.
5. Ipp E, Dobbs RE, Harris V, Arimura A, Vale W and Unger RH: The effects of gastrin, gastric inhibitory polypeptide, secretin, and the octopeptide of cholecystokinin upon immunoreactive somatostatin release by the perfused canine pancreas. J Clin Invest. 60 (1977) 1216-1219.
6. Kaneto A, Kosaka K and Nakao K: Effects of stimulation of the vagus nerve on insulin secretion. Endocrinology 80 (1967) 530-536.
7. Kaneto A, Miki E and Kosaka K: Effects of vagal stimulation on glucagon and insulin secretion. Endocrinology 95 (1974) 1005-1010.
8. Kaneto A, Miki E and Kosaka K: Effect of Beta and B_2 Adrenoreceptor stimulants infused intrapancreatically on glucagon and insulin secretion. Endocrinology 97 (1975) 1166-1173.
9. King BM, Bauta AR, Tharell GN, Bruce BK and Frohman LA: Hypothalamic hyperinsulinemia and obesity: a role of adrenal glucocorticoids. Am J Physiol. 245 (1983) E194-199.
10. Kolb B and Nonneman AJ: Prefrontal cortex and the regulation of food intake in the rat. J comp physiol Psychol. 89 (1975) 806-815.
11. Leibowitz SF, Hammer NJ and Chang K: Feeding behavior induced by central norepinephrine injection is attenuated by discrete lesions in the hypothalamic paraventricular nucleus. Pharmacol Biochem and Behav. 19 (1983) 945-951.
12. Luiten PGM and Room P: Interrelations between lateral, dorsomedial and ventromedial hypothalamic nuclei in the rat. An HRP study. Brain Res. 190 (1980) 321-332.
13. Luiten PGM, Koolhaas JM, De Boer S and Koopmans SJ: The corticomedial amygdala in the central nervous system organization of agonistic behavior. Brain Res. 332 (1985) 283-297.
14. Luiten PGM, Ter Horst GJ, Karst H and Steffens AB: The course of paraventricular hypothalamic efferents to autonomic structures in medulla and spinal cord. Brain Res. 329 (1985) 374-378.
15. Luiten PGM, Ter Horst GJ, Koopmans SJ, Rietberg M and Steffens AB: Preganglionic innervation of the pancreas islet cells in the rat. J Auton nerv Syst. 10 (1984) 27-42.
16. McCaleb ML, Myers RD, Singer G and Willis G: Hypothalamic norepinephrine in the rat during feeding and push-pull perfusion with glucose, 2 DG, or insulin. Am J Physiol. 236 (1979) R312-321.
17. Merchenthaler J, Hynes MA, Vigh S, Schally AV and Petrusz P: Corticotropin releasing factor (CRF). Origin and course of afferent pathways to the median eminence (ME) of the rat hypothalamus. Neuroendocrinology 39 (1984) 296-306.
18. Müller WA, Faloona GR and Unger RH: The effect of alanine on glucagon secretion. J Clin Invest. 50 (1971) 2215-2218.
19. Olivier B: Behavioral Functions of the Medial Hypothalamus in the Rat. Doctoral Thesis, University of Groningen, 1977.

20. Oomura Y: Glucose as a regulator of neuronal activity. In: Advances in Metabolic Disorders. CNS Regulation of Carbohydrate Metabolism, New York: Academic Press (1983) Vol. 10 p 31-65.
21. Porte D, Jr: A receptor mechanism for the inhibition of insulin release by epinephrine in man. J Clin Invest. 46 (1967) 86-94.
22. Porte D, Jr: Beta adrenergic stimulation of insulin release in man. Diabetes 16 (1967) 150-155.
23. Schmitt P, Abou-Hamed H et Karli P: Effects aversifs et appétitifs induits par stimulation mésencéphalique et hypothalamique. Brain Res. 130 (1977) 521-530.
24. Sclafani A, Belluzi JG and Grossman SP: Effects of lesions in the hypothalamus and amygdala on feeding behavior in the rat. J comp physiol Psychol. 72 (1970) 394-403.
25. Shimazu T: Reciprocal innervation of the liver: its significance in metabolic control. In: Advances in Metabolic Disorders. Regulation of Carbohydrate Metatolism. New York: Academic Press (1983) Vol. 10 p 355-384.
26. Steffens AB: The influence of the oral cavity on the release of insulin in the rat. Am J Physiol. 230 (1976) 1411-1415.
27. Steffens AB: The modulatory effect of the hypothalamus on glucagon and insulin secretion in the rat. Diabetologia 20 (1981) 411-416.
28. Steffens AB, Damsma G, van der Gugten J and Luiten PGM: Circulating free fatty acids, insulin, and glucose during chemical stimulation of hypothalamus in rats. Am J Physiol. 247 (1984) E765-771.
29. Steffens AB, Flik G, Kuipers F, Lotter EC and Luiten PGM: Hypothalamically induced insulin release and its potentiation during oral and intravenous glucose loads. Brain Res. 301 (1984) 351-361.
30. Strubbe JH and van Wachem P: Insulin secretion by the transplanted neonatal pancreas during food intake in fasted and fed rats. Diabetologia 20 (1981) 228-236.
31. Ter Horst GJ, Luiten PGM and Kuipers F: Descending pathways from hypothalamus to dorsal motor vagus and ambiguus nuclei in the rat. J auton nerv Syst. 11 (1984) 59-75.
32. Ter Horst GJ, Groenewegen HJ, Karst H and Luiten PGM: Phaseolus vulgaris leuco-agglutinin immunohistochemistry. A comparison between autoradiographic and lectin tracing of neuronal efferents. Brain Res. 307 (1984) 379-383.
33. Torres-Aleman I, Mason-Garcia M and Schally AV: Stimulation of insulin secretion by corticotropin-releasing factor (CRF) in anesthetized rats. Peptides 5 (1984) 541-546.
34. Van der Gugten J and Slangen JL: Release of endogenous catecholamines from the rat hypothalamus related to feeding and other behaviors. Pharmacol Biochem Behav. 7 (1977) 211-219.
35. Yoshimatsu H, Niijima A, Oomura Y, Yamabe K and Katafuchi T: Effects of hypothalamic lesion on pancreatic autonomic nerve activity in the rat. Brain Res. 303 (1984) 147-152.

1.2.5. Cellular insulin resistance
Tj. Wieringa

INTRODUCTION
    In the last decade it has become increasingly clear that cellular
insulin resistance is an important feature of type I and type II
diabetes mellitus. The most frequently quoted definition of insulin
resistance is the one proposed by Berson and Yalow (1). They define
insulin resistance as "a state in which increased amounts of insulin
are required to elicit a quantitatively normal response". However, the
experimental data obtained elucidate that a quantitatively normal
response is often not achieved, even at supra-physiological concentrations of insulin. In an attempt to clarify the confusion
generated by the use of various definitions Kahn (2) recently defined
insulin resistance as "a state in which a normal concentration of
insulin produces a less than normal biological response". A consequence of this definition is that even a 'normal' metabolic state,
such as fasting, can now be regarded as insulin resistance.
    On the cellular level insulin resistance states may be divided into
those due to a decreased sensitivity for insulin, those due to a decrease in maximal response to insulin and those which are combinations
of changes in sensitivity and in responsiveness. This distinction is
important since the molecular mechanisms that produce these various
forms of insulin resistance may be quite different. Therefore a
detailed knowledge of insulin binding to its receptor, of the cellular
processing of the insulin-receptor complex and of the regulation of
the insulin-sensitive pathways in intracellular metabolism is required
for the evaluation of the defects of insulin action in clinical disorders
of glucose tolerance .

Dose-response relationship
    When insulin acts on target cells, it does not activate a single
process but it rather regulates various biochemical events within the
cells. This complexity is one of the reasons why the mechanism of
insulin action has not yet been elucidated so many years after the
discovery of insulin.
    The regulating role of insulin on the blood glucose concentration
is not only an effect of the stimulation of the uptake and oxidation of
glucose, the synthesis of glycogen and lipid from glucose, but also of
the inhibiting effects on glycogenolysis, gluconeogenesis and lipolysis.
In addition, the effects of insulin vary both in time course and dose-
response. For instance stimulation of glucose transport occurs within
seconds after hormone binding, whereas the expression of the effects
on most cytoplasmic enzymes requires minutes to hours.

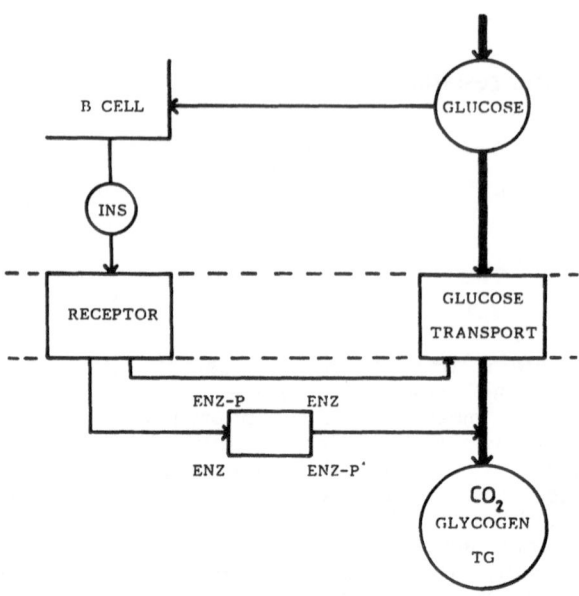

The first step in insulin action (see figure) is specific binding of the hormone to its membrane receptor. This interaction is associated with the generation or activation of a chemical mediator or perhaps mediators yielding changes in the degree of phosphorylation of several key enzymes of glucose and fat metabolism and to an increase in glucose uptake in muscle and fat tissue. Thus the major function of insulin or glucose metabolism is in fact to accelerate or to decelerate various biochemical pathways and not, as is often assumed, to switch on or off enzyme reactions.

The simplest assumption is a 1:1 relation between receptor occupancy and the final biological response. However, for most insulin-receptor systems maximal response is seen by concentrations of insulin by which only a small proportion of the receptors is occupied. Further increase in receptor occupancy does not increase the biological response. It seems that many receptors have no effect and are "spare". Roth and Grunfeld (3) argue however, that none of the receptors are spare, but that all are used. A measured receptor occupancy of 10% means that all the receptors are occupied 10% of the time. Moreover the degree of spareness does not seem to be determined by the absolute number or the concentration of receptors, but to depend on the ratio of the receptors to capacity of the events which will respond. In fact it means that the degree of spareness of receptors in a single cell varies if one response or another response is measured. The functional consequence of the "spare-receptor" concept is that we can distinguish in the dose-response relationship sensitivity and responsiveness.

A decrease in affinity is expressed in the dose-response curve as a shift towards higher insulin concentrations. The maximal response can be achieved, but higher insulin concentrations are needed to obtain the same effect. The sensitivity for insulin has decreased. This can be seen when the number of receptors is reduced in a system in which receptors exceed the responding systems. In contrast a defect in one of the post-binding events in insulin action or in the effector system itself produces a decrease in maximal response that cannot be overcome by a further increase in concentration of insulin. This is a decreased responsiveness.

In the last years much attention has been given to detect changes in cellular action of insulin in obesity and diabetes. Many studies were performed in vitro with cells isolated from experimental animals. We will focus on changes in binding capacity and post-binding events.

Changes in insulin binding

We are familiar with the observation that the plasma insulin concentration fluctuates widely in response to changes within the body. With the introduction of methods to measure directly the binding of insulin to its receptors it became clear that the concentration of receptors at the cell surface also changes rapidly in response to signals from inside and outside the cell. A dynamic situation exists in which receptors continuously flow to and from the surface of the cell. Often an inverse relation is found between the chronic level of insulin and the cell surface receptor number. Thus the higher the hormone levels, the lower the receptor concentration. The process involved is induced by the hormone and is referred to as "downregulation" and seems to be specific for peptide hormones in general. The molecular mechanism by which "downregulation" occurs is not known in detail but includes aggregation of hormone-receptor complex in specific vesicles, internalization and degradation by lysosomes. This can be associated with or without effects on "de novo" receptor biosynthesis and/or insertion into the membrane (4).

In most obese persons the plasma insulin concentrations are higher than in normal persons irrespective of glucose tolerance. These observations suggest a decrease in sensitivity with the possibility that this change is caused by a reduction in number of receptors. "Downregulation" was found in these persons, but it is a matter of debate if this proves a causal relationship between a reduced number of cell surface receptors induced by hyperinsulinaemia and insulin resistance.

Both affinity and receptor number are directly regulated by insulin. Other hormones that affect insulin receptors are growth hormone, which changes mainly receptor concentration and glucocorticoids which change mainly receptor affinity. Binding is very sensitive to changes in pH and diet. Diets with a high content of carbohydrates and fat reduce cell surface receptor concentration, but dietary fiber, both soluble and insoluble, increase insulin binding. Moreover insulin binding increases through excercise both acutely and 'chronically'. Oral hypoglycemic drugs have been reported to increase cell surface receptor concentration.

Post-binding changes

a) The insulin receptor

Over the past few years studies have suggested that the insulin receptor is composed of two subunits a α-subunit (mol. weight

125.000 D) and a β-subunit (90.000 D).

These subunits are derived from a single precursor. Usually the receptor is found as a disulfide-linked complex composed of 2α and 2β-subunits. Covalent cross-linking of radioactive insulin to its receptor has shown that the α-subunit probably forms the insulin binding site. The β-subunit appears to be the effector portion of the receptor and shows increased phosphorylation of one or more tyrosines after the receptor-hormone complex is formed (5). However, in intact cells and in immunoprecipitated receptor preparations, insulin stimulated phosphorylation of serine residues (6,7). Possibly, the two phosphorylation states represents functional differences. The autophosphorylation of the insulin receptor increases its activity to function as a phosphotransferase towards several exogenous substrates. How far the receptor autophosphorylation or receptor kinase activity play a role in translation of the signal remains to be established. An interesting aspect of tyrosine kinase activity of the insulin receptor is that membrane receptors for growth factors which have some insulin like effects are also hormone-responsive tyrosine kinases (5).

The amino-acid sequence of both the receptor for insulin and for human epidermal growth factor (EGF) has recently been determined (5,8,9). However, no overall similarity between the sequence of the cytoplasmic portion of the β-chain was found, although there are several obvious analogies. Both show within the tyrosine kinase domain partial homology with receptors to oncogenes. The insulin receptor has partial homology with products of the members of the socalled SRC oncogene family, and the EGF receptor with V-erb-B oncogene products.

It will be interesting to test whether the corresponding regions of the insulin and EGF receptor genes are oncogenic.

Defects in insulin receptor autophosphorylation were found in cells taken from a patient with a type A syndrome of severe insulin resistance and acanthosis nigricans, in which the insulin concentration increases up to 1000 times the normal level in order to produce normal glucose levels (10). Despite normal or near normal insulin binding, the receptor showed 50% decrease in insulin stimulated autophosphorylation. In parallel the receptor showed a 40% decrease in phosphotransferase activities. The defects were both present in freshly isolated cells and in cells in long-term culture, suggesting that the defects are genetic in nature.

In experimental animals various forms of insulin resistance can be seen. In genetically obese animals or when obesity is experimentally induced insulin resistance is seen both in vivo and in vitro.
The resistance cannot be explained by a decrease in receptor number. It is supposed that a change in an early post binding event is responsible for the impaired action of insulin. In muscles of insulin resistant obese mice the insulin receptor phosphotransferase activity is markedly decreased (11). A causal relationship was found between resistance and impaired phosphotransferase activity. Similarly, it has been shown that insulin resistance, which occur in streptozotocin-induced diabetes in rats, is accompanied by a decreased kinase activity of liver receptors (12). However, in other studies on experimental induced diabetes, no change in liver receptor autophosphorylation was observed (13). In contrast, even increased insulin

stimulated autophosphorylation was found (14).

b) Signal translation
Despite detailed knowledge regarding hormone-receptor interaction, knowledge concerning signalling is minimal. The question how the information of the insulin-receptor association is transformed into a biological response still remains open. Different mechanisms have been proposed. A second messenger or a chemical mediator, that alters cell function by regulation of enzyme activity, is still the most attractive hypothesis. Enzyme regulation by phosphorylation and dephosphorylation has been widely investigated and various enzymes in glucose metabolism regulated their activity in this way. Whether these studies have potential clinical significance remains to be established.

c) Glucose uptake
One of insulin's major biological effects is the stimulation of glucose uptake. Abnormalities of this aspect in insulin action can lead to important clinical and pathophysiological states. Glucose uptake occurs via specific proteins located in the plasma membrane. Two groups have recently reported that the glucose transport units in the cell are in two pools, one (functional) is in the plasma membrane and another (not functional) is somewhere intracellular (15,16). Insulin causes a translocation of the transport units from the non-functional to the functional pool. There seems little doubt that an increase in the number of functional transport units is a major effect of insulin in adipocytes and in muscle, but criticism has been raised. This hypothesis cannot explain all the effects of insulin. Moreover the transfer of units from the intracellular pool to the plasma membrane must be surprisingly rapid, since the maximal effect of insulin on glucose uptake is observed within 1 minute. Nevertheless the translocation hypothesis fits with the data obtained thusfar with cells from obese and diabetic subjects.

In experimental diabetes and in fasting the ability of insulin to stimulate glucose transport in adipocytes is markedly reduced (17-19). Recent studies suggest that this is associated with a depletion of transport units in the intracellular pool and in the reduction in the ability of insulin to stimulate the translocation of the units to the plasma membrane. Using an organ culture system for adipose tissue or cell culture most studies indicate that sulfonylureas and biguanides potentiate the stimulating effects of insulin on hexose transport at submaximal and maximal effective concentrations of insulin. It will therefore be interesting to test whether or not oral hypoglycemic drugs potentiate translocation of the transport units and eventually will normalize glucose uptake in cells from diabetic subjects.

Summarizing the in vitro data at present, we may say that although numerous factors influence receptor number and affinity, the contribution of the abnormalities in insulin binding account for only a small part for the impaired action of insulin. However, postbinding defects especially in the effector system (glucose metabolism) itself, contribute to a large extent to the impaired action of insulin found in obesity and diabetes. But the interpretation of in vitro studies is relatively simple. In vivo the situation is more complex. Not all the target cells are exposed to the same concentration of insulin. Some cell types are more responsive than others. Moreover within a single cell type some processes are more sensitive to insulin than others.

Further a particular pathway may become unresponsive while other pathways remain sensitive to insulin. Thus when measuring a dose-response relation in order to detect the location of defects in insulin action, we must realize that the curve obtained consists of various processes and that changes in these processes contribute to a different extent to the overall change in dose-response relation.

For dose-response curves in vivo various techniques are used. Insulin and glucose can be continuously infused while endogenous insulin secretion is inhibited by an infusion of adrenaline and propranolol or somotostatin. Different rates of insulin infusion were used to establish dose-response curves. Another technique is the 'euglycemic clamp' technique. In this technique glucose uptake is measured at various levels of constant plasma insulin concentrations.

Studies in humans thusfar indicate that carbohydrate intolerance increases when post-binding defects in peripheral tissues dominate. It is not clear which factors mediate these defects in insulin action and if they are the primary defects or are secondary to hypoinsulinemia (20).

REFERENCES

1. Berson SA, and Yalow RS: Insulin 'antagonists' and insulin resis-
    tance. In: Diabetes Mellitus: Theory and Practice. Ellenberg M,
    Rifkin H. McGraw-Hill, New York, 1970, 388-423.

2. Kahn CR: Insulin resistance, insulin insensitivity, insulin un-
    responsiveness: A necessary distinction. Metabolism, 27, 1978,
    1893-1902.

3. Roth J, Grunfeld C: Endocrine Systems: Mechanisms of Disease,
    Target Cells and Receptors. (Chapter 2) In: Textbook of
    Endocrinology (6th ed.), Williams RH. W.B. Saunders Company
    Philadelphia, 1981, 15-72.

4. Posner BI, Bergeron JJM, Josefsberg Z, et al.: Polypeptide
    Hormones: intracellular receptors and internalization. Rec. Prog.
    Horm. Res., 37, 1981, 539-582.

5. Ullrich A, Bell JR, Chen EY, et al.: Human insulin receptor and
    its relation to the tyrosine kinase family of oncogenes. Nature,
    313, 1985, 756-761.

6. Kasuga M, Zick Y, Blithe DL, Karlsson FA, Häring HU, Kahn CR:
    Insulin stimulation of phosphorylation of the β-subunit of the
    insulin receptor. Formation of both phosphoserine and phospho-
    tyrosine. J. Biol. Chem., 257, 1982, 9891-9894.

7. Gazzano H, Kowalski A, Fehlman M, Van Obberghen E: Two different
    protein-kinase activities are associated with the insulin receptor.
    Biochem. J., 216, 1983, 575-582.

8. Ullrich A, Coussens L, Hayflick JS, et al.: Human epidermal
    growth factor receptor cDNA sequence and aberrant expression of
    the amplified gene in A 431 epidermoid carcinoma cells. Nature,
    309, 1984, 418-425.

9. Downward J, Yarden Y, Mayes E, et al.: Close similarity of epi-
    dermal growth factor receptor and V-erb-B oncogene protein
    sequences. Nature, 307, 1984, 521-527.

10. Grigorescu F, Flier JS. Kahn CR: Defect in insulin receptor
    phosphorylation in erythrocytes and fibroblasts associated with
    severe insulin resistance. J. Biol. Chem., 259, 1984, 15003-
    15006.

11. Le Marchand-Brustel Y, Grémeaux T, Ballotti R, Van Obberghen
    E: Insulin receptor tyrosine kinase is defective in skeletal muscle
    of insulin-resistant obese mice. Nature, 315, 1985, 676-679.

12. Kadowaki T, Kasuga M, Akannura Y, Ezaki O, Takaku F: Decreased
    autophosphorylation of the insulin receptor-kinase in strepto-
    zotocin-diabetic rats. J. Biol. Chem., 259, 1984, 14208-14216.

13. Amatruda JM, Roncone AM: Normal hepatic insulin receptor auto-phosphorylation in non-ketoticdiabetes mellitus. Biochem. Biophys. Res. Commun., 129, 1985, 163-170.

14. Blackshear PJ, Nemenoff RA, Avruch J: Characteristics of insulin and epidermal growth factor stimulation of receptor auto-phosphorylation in detergent extracts of rat liver and transplantable rat hepatomas. Endocrinology, 114, 1981, 141-152.

15. Suzuki K, Kono T: Evidence that insulin causes translocation of glucose transport activity to the plasma membrane from an intra-cellular storage site. Proc. Natl. Acad. Sci, USA, 77, 1980, 2542-2545.

16. Cushman SW, Wardzala LJ: Potential mechanism of insulin action on glucose transport in isolated rat adipose cell. J. Biol. Chem., 255, 1980, 4758-4762.

17. Kasuga M, Akanuma Y, Iwamoto Y, Kosaka K: Insulin binding and glucose metabolism in adipocytes of steptozotocin-diabetic rats. Am. J. Physiol., 4, 1978, E175-E182.

18. Wieringa Tj, Krans HMJ: Reduced glucose transport and in-creased binding of insulin in adipocytes from diabetic and fasted rats. Biochim. Biophys. Acta, 538, 1978, 563-570.

19. Kobayashi M, Olefsky JM: Effects of streptozotocin-induced diabetes on insulin binding, glucose transport, and intracellular glucose metabolism in isolated rat adipocytes. Diabetes, 28, 1979, 87-95.

20. Reaven GM, Chen YI, Coulston AM, et al.: Insulin secretion and action in non-insulin-dependent diabetes mellitus. Is insulin resistance secondary to hypoinsulinemia? Am. J. Med., 75, (Suppl. 5B), 1983, 85-93.

2. Treatment of Diabetes Mellitus

2.1. Diet and hypoglycaemic agents

2.1.1. Introduction: Diet and hypoglycaemic agents
J.L. Touber

Dietary advice for the diabetic individual has shown a remarkable change over the last decade. In the past the dietary rules always began with 'thou shalt not eat' followed by a long list of foodstuffs, which were largely ignored by the patients except for the highly neurasthenic ones. Recently however, prestigious diabetologists recommend a dietary regime, which differs only marginally -if at all- from the nutritional program advocated for the general population, viz. the so called 'prudent diet' (high in carbohydrate, low in cholesterol and saturated fats). The American Diabetes Association and other venerated institutions have even begun to lift the ban on sucrose and alcohol, and one may ask whether there are any dietary rules left which apply specifically for the diabetic individual. However, despite the emancipation of the 'diabetes diet', there still are.

The primary objective of the nutritional program for the diabetic subject is the control of blood glucose and lipid levels. In the youngster with insulin-dependent diabetes (type I) normal growth and development by adequate nutrition intake takes precedence over rigid and rigorous control of blood glucose levels. 'Normalization' of blood glucose - that is avoidance of overt or symptomatic hyper-and hypoglycaemia - is aimed at by the proper timing and spacing of meals in relation to the insulin injections.

In the overweight type II diabetic subject the emphasis is on the normalization of weight, with the attendant improvement in glucose and lipid metabolism. If a type II patient is on hypoglycaemic therapy (insulin, oral agents) spacing of meals becomes mandatory.

In both type I and type II patients the dietary program should be appropriate, that is (apart from being nutritionally adequate) it should be
based on the preference of the patient and his or her family; the composition and the quality of the diet (if not the quantity and / or the
spacing)should also be applicable to the family members.

As noted before, the dietary advice for both type I and II diabetic subjects is not different from that recommended for the general population
with respect to the quality and quantity of proteins and fats, nor is
there a difference in the quantity of carbohydrates (50-60% of the total
calories). There are, however, differences of opinion and uncertainties
with respect to the quality of the carbohydrates.

The American Diabetes Association has recently issued a policy statement, in which the consumption of 'a modest amount' of sucrose and more
emphasis on carbohydrate containing foods that produce the smallest
rise in blood sugar, is advocated. This advice seems odd, because many
respected diabetologists insist on the avoidance (or at least reduction)
of rapidly absorbed simple sugars. There is, however, evidence that some
commonly used foods containing complex carbohydrates (bread, potatoes)
raise the blood sugar as quickly as glucose or sucrose, while other
foods (e.g. beans) cause more moderate glycaemic excursions. As pointed
out by Josse and Jenkins in this book,   'the glycaemic index' of
starchy foods is not simply related to their fiber content, but also to
the physiological characteristics of the starch involved, both before
and after preparation of the meal. Although more emphasis on 'lente'
carbohydrates is clearly valuable (for both the diabetic and the non-
diabetic individual), it seems unlikely that the diabetic population in
the Netherlands will ever switch 'en masse' from bread and potatoes to
beans, corn, rice and spaghetti (cooked 'aldente').

If the ADA recommendations are accepted by the medical profession, we
could probably do away with the artificial sweeteners (saccharin, cycla-
mate, xylitol,sorbitol, aspartame) and with the so- called 'foodstuffs
for diabetes patients' (jams, chocolate, soft drinks, etc.) containing
these products.

Although it is quite clear that type II diabetes is a disorder associa-

ted with the 'Westernization' of nutrition, it should not be forgotten
that it is also associated with lack of physical activity which is typical of the western life-style. Dr. Elliott P. Joslin taught us that exercise is of great help in the treatment of diabetes and that it should be
employed in each and every case. He quoted one of his wisest diabetics,
Major W., case 352, who said: "First, it is very hard to start the exercise, and the less one feels inclined to start, the more one needs it.
Second, it is neither necessary nor desirable that it should be violent.
I found a quiet ride of an hour, walking or jogging after taking some-
thing on the stomach, started up my old metabolism for the whole day".
Bogardus et al.(1984) have recently compared the effects of physical
training in addition to hypocaloric diet in type II diabetics with the
effects of diet therapy alone. They found that in both groups the improvement in fasting plasma glucose and meal tolerance appeared to be
attributable mostly to a decrease in basal endogenous glucose production,
with an increased hepatic sensitivity to insulin. However, the trained
group had a significantly greater increase in apparent carbohydrate
storage rates in comparison with the untrained group, and therefore diet
therapy plus physical training produced a more significant approach
toward normal.

With regard to the hypoglycaemic agents, the issue is still clouded by
the strife and controversy stirred up by the findings of the University
Group Diabetes Program study. It seems impossible to resolve this
controversy.

The UGDP study tried to answer the question whether or not control of
blood glucose levels (using diet plus insulin, tolbutamide, phenformin
or placebo) would prevent or delay the vascular complications of type
II diabetics. The findings provided no evidence that insulin (given in
a fixed or in a variable dosis), or the other drugs used will alter the
course of the vascular complications.

The disappointing failure to observe beneficial effects of hypoglycaemic
therapy was, however, not what caused the medical community to erupt
into the 'tolbutamide controversy', a controversy probably without
parallel in modern medicine.

The main reason for this was that the UGDP findings also suggested (but did not prove - the study was not designed to that end) that the oral agents might be less effective than diet alone or than diet plus insulin in prolonging life, because an increase in cardiovascular mortality was found in the subjects treated with oral agents. This raised the possibility that long term use of oral agents, apart from being ineffective, might even be harmful.

Today, 25 years after the inception of the UGDP trial, we are still not sure whether good (or even tight) control of blood glucose will prevent or delay the micro- and / or macrovascular complications of diabetes. (UGDP, 1982, Siperstein, 1983). The fact that on both sides of the Atlantic large trials are under way to reexamine the issue (NIH clinical trial, 1982, UK prospective study, 1983), exemplifies our basal ignorance. Unfortunately, the results cannot be expected before well into the nineties. What then is our therapeutic strategy in the interim ?

Since type I diabetes is characterized by insulin deficiency, it is clear that all type I patients should be treated with insulin. Insulin therapy is also mandatory in women with gestational diabetes. How tight the blood sugar control should be, is largely dictated by the circumstances of the individual patient; much more emphasis on normoglycaemia is needed in a young, pregnant woman than in an elderly lady.

The real problem, of course, is what to do with the 80% of all diabetic subjects belonging to the type II category. In theory at least, we all agree that these patients should first and foremost change their lifestyle with emphasis on diet and exercise. If a strict regime fails to control hyperglycaemia sufficiently (the degree of control strived for again varying from patient to patient, vide supra) and the patient is symptomatic, or has acute or chronic complications (diabetic or non - diabetic), hypoglycaemic therapy is needed. In all these cases, I would prescribe insulin, because insulin is safer (Prout, 1975).

The indication for treatment with hypoglycaemic agents (insulin or tablets) in all other type II diabetics (viz. the relatively mild diabetic, who is relatively young and healthy), remains dubious. Ten years

ago an editorial (Lancet, 1975) on the merits and demerits of the oral
hypoglycaemic agents prophecied: "Surely now there will be an end to the
gross overprescription of these drugs for elderly patients with mild
diabetes, for whom a proper diet that they can understand and adhere
to is the only necessary treatment. At the very least, the UGDP has
performed an immense service if physicians are thereby persuaded that
the time taken to construct and explain an appropriate diet in
diabetes is indeed a better investment of their skill than the instant
prescription of a potent and potentially dangerous drug".

It is, however, quite clear that the gross overprescription of oral
agents has not ended, because there are marked differences in utilization of these drugs between different countries without evidence of
equally marked differences in the incidence of diabetes (Bergman et al.
1979, see also Keen and Ng Tang Fui in this   book   ). It is equally
clear that non-medical forces in the marketplace for medical care in our
overmedicated society must be held responsible for this phenomenon - it
should be realized that the potential market for these drugs is close to
one or even two percent of the total population.

Regardless of whether we wish to emphasize or discount the evidence for
a relationship between an increased cardiovascular mortality and therapy with oral agents, we must realize that some of the adverse effects
of these drugs, viz. hypoglycaemia and lactic acidosis carry a very high
mortality (10 and 50%, respectively). Nor is it safe to assume that
these cases are rare and can be prevented anyway by avoiding overdosage.

The Swedish adverse drug reactions advisory committee (Böttiger et al.
1979) reported that the oral antidiabetic drugs headed the list of drugs
implicated as a cause of death in Sweden, while Asplund et al. (1983)
after analysis of 57 cases of glibenclamide associated hypoglycaemia
reported to the Swedish committee (10 patients died), concluded that
the 57 patients probably represented only a minority of all hypoglycaemic episodes caused by glibenclamide.

With regard to overdosage, it should be noted that Berger (1971) showed
that in 95% of the casualties of oral agents in Switzerland a correct

dosis had in fact been prescribed, and Asplund et al.(1983) concluded that neither the absence of apparent contributing factors (e.g. hepatic and / or renal impairment, alcohol, drug interactions, etc.) nor low dosage of glibenclamide precludes the occurrence of serious hypoglycaemia. The vagaries of therapy with the oral agents may - in part - be explained by the findings of Scott and Poffenbarger (1979), who demonstrated that the rate of tolbutamide disposal is under genetic control (resulting in rapid or slow inactivation). Other pharmacokinetic studies have shown extremely large interindividual variations in serum levels of tolbutamide, chlorpropamide and glibenclamide, without a correlation between the dose administered and the plasma level (Melander et al.,1978; Sartor et. al, 1980; Bergman et al.,1980).

Therefore in the treatment of those type II diabetics in whom hypoglycaemic therapy is really deemed necessary, the unpredictable pharmacokinetics of the oral agents, together with the likelihood of drug interactions (resulting from acute changes in protein binding) favours the choice of the safest hypoglycaemic agent presently available: insulin.

REFERENCES

- American Diabetes Association: Policy Statement 'Glycemic effects of carbohydrates'.
  Diabetes Care,7: 607-608, 1984.
- Bogardus C, Ravussin E, Robbins DC, Wolfe RR, Horton ES and Sims EAH: Effects of physical training and diet therapy on carbohydrate metabolism in patients with glucose intolerance and non-insulin-dependent diabetes mellitus.
  Diabetes, 33: 311-318, 1984.
- University Group Diabetes Program: Effects of hypoglycemic agents on vascular complications in patients with adult onset diabetes. VIII. Evaluation of insulin therapy: final report.
  Diabetes, 31: suppl. 5, 1-81, 1982.
- Siperstein MD: Diabetic microangiopathy and the control of blood glucose.
  New Engl.J.Med., 309: 1577-1579, 1983.
- NIH proposed protocol for the clinical trial to assess the relationship between metabolic control and the early vascular complications of insulin-dependent diabetes.
  Diabetes 31, 1132-1133, 1982.
- UK Prospective study of therapies of maturity-onset diabetes.
  I. Effects of diet, sulphonylurea, insulin   biguanide therapy on fasting plasma glucose and body weight over one year.
  Diabetologia, 24: 404-411, 1983.
- Prout TE: A progress report on the University Group Diabetes Program.
  Int.J.Clin.Pharmacol., 12: 244-246, 1975.
- Editorial: Oral hypoglycaemics in diabetes mellitus.
  Lancet, ii: 48, 1975.
- Bergman U: International comparisons of drug utilization: use of anti-diabetic drugs in seven European countries.
  In: Studies of drug-utilization. WHO Regional European Series, 147-162, 1979.
- Böttiger LE, Furhoff AK and Holmberg L: Fatal reactions to drugs: a 10-year material from the Swedish adverse drug reactions committee.
  Acta Med.Scand., 205: 451-458, 1979.

- Asplund K, Wiholm BE and Lithner F: Glibenclamide-associated hypo-
glycaemia: a report on 57 cases.
Diabetologia, 24: 412-417, 1983.
- Berger W: 88 Schwere hypoglykämiezwischenfalle unter den Behandlung
mit Sulfonylharnstoffen.
Schweiz.Med.Wschr., 71: 1013-1016, 1971.
- Scott J and Poffenberger PL: Pharmacogenetics of tolbutamide metabo-
lism in humans.
Diabetes, 28: 41-46, 1979.
- Melander A, Sartor G, Wahlin E, Schersten B, Bitzen PO: Serum tolbuta-
mide and chlorporpamide concentrations in patients with diabetes
mellitus.
Brit.Med.J., i: 142-144, 1978.
- Sartor G, Melander A, Schersten B, Wahlin-Boll E: Serum glibenclamide
in diabeic patients and influence of food on the kinetics and effects
of glibenclamide.
Diabetologia, 18: 17-22, 1980.
- Bergman V, Christenson I, Jansson B, Wiholm BE, Ostman J: Wide varia-
tions in serum chlorpropamide concentrations among outpatients.
Eur.J.Clin.Pharmacol., 18: 165-169, 1980.

2.1.2. Diet and Diabetes

R.G. Josse, A.L. Jenkins and D.J.A. Jenkins

1. INTRODUCTION

Over the last 2 millenia there have been great differences of opinion on the diets which should be prescribed for diabetic patients. Two thousand years ago Indian physicians advocated high carbohydrate diets rich in unprocessed cereals and legumes for the treatment of type II diabetes. By the time of Allen, just prior to the discovery of insulin, low carbohydrate, hypocaloric diets were being used. With the advent of the insulin, although less emphasis was placed on diet, carbohydrate restriction tended to persist despite the studies of Himsworth indicating the possible value of increased carbohydrate intake.

The possible value of higher carbohydrate intakes in terms of the lipid lowering effect was later demonstrated by Connor and Stone[1] in long-term studies although this effect has not always been confirmed.[2] Furthermore Brunzell and coworkers demonstrated in patients with carbohydrate intolerance that glucose tolerance was improved on very high carbohydrate formula diets.[3]

Most recently a move to increase the carbohydrate content of the diabetic diet has been prompted by concern over high fat intakes and increased risk of cardiovascular disease to which the diabetic is already particularly prone. Evidence which favours the active reduction of blood lipids[4-6] continues to accumulate. In view of this, many diabetes Associations have revised their dietary guidelines by recommending that fat intake be reduced, the P/S ratio increased and that carbohydrate intake be increased to approximately 50% of total calories.[7-9] In this way the diabetic diet also reflects the dietary advice given by the Heart Foundations. The rationale for the recommendations have already been well stated by the Nutrition Sub-Committee of the British Diabetic Association[9] and most recently by the American Diabetes Association.[10]

Such advice has also focussed attention on the possible differences between individual carbohydrate foods and the consequences of increasing their use in the diet. Early on insulins were developed with different time-courses of activity (e.g. regular and lente). Although it was also acknowledged that insulin action should follow the pattern of carbohydrate intake little attention was actually paid to potential differences between carbohydrates. With the advent of interest in dietary fiber this changed. It was demonstrated that even unabsorbable materials within the gastrointestinal tract could influence rate of nutrient absorption, endocrine responses and hence metabolic events.

Early on it was demonstrated that purified viscous fibers such as guar added to test meals flattened the glycemic response and also the insulin response.[11] (Fig 1 Lancet 1976) When incorporated into foods in metabolic diets they resulted in reduced urinary glucose[12] and ketone body outputs [13] and improved diabetic control could be demonstrated in long term outpatient studies [14-16](Fig 2 - long term guar).

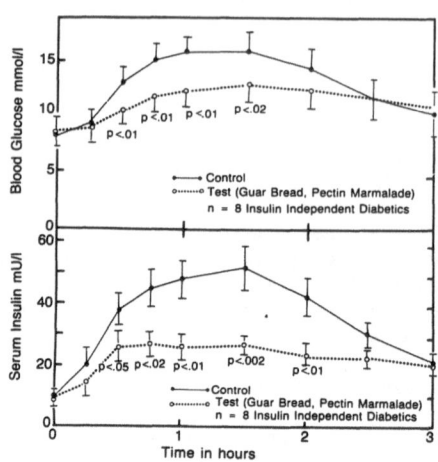

FIGURE 1. Effect on postprandial levels of glucose and insulin in eight non-insulin-requiring diabetics of adding 16g guar to bread and 10g pectin to the marmalade in a test-meal breakfast containing 106g carbohydrate.[11]

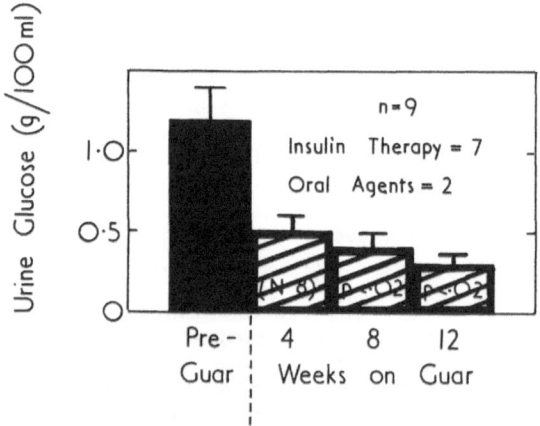

FIGURE 2. Urine glucose concentration of nine diabetic patients both before and during 12 weeks of taking guar crispbread.[14]

At the same time studies by Anderson using high fiber high carbohydrate diets[17-19] indicated that such diets resulted in good diabetic control which could be achieved even in the face of a gradual reduction in insulin dosage (Fig 3 Anderson). Indeed, in patients taking relatively small amounts of insulin this could be gradually reduced and withdrawn altogether despite a lack of major change in body weight. Such diets have proved useful in the long term management of diabetes.

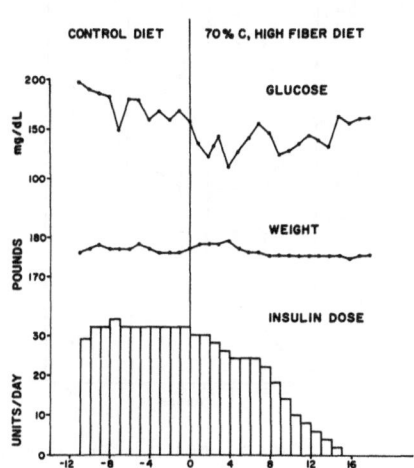

FIGURE 3. Fasting blood glucose, body weight and insulin dose in a diabetic man on control (43%) carbohydrate low fiber and high carbohydrate (70%), high fiber diet.[19]

These diets were not only high in fiber but contained foods which were subsequently shown to liberate their products of digestion at a reduced rate. It was also shown that these rates of digestion related well to the glycemic response produced following ingestion of the food. The term lente carbohydrate was therefore coined for foods which were slowly digested, released their products of digestion slowly into the circulation and caused flatter, more sustained elevations of the blood glucose.

2. FIBER

2.1. Physiological Effects of Fiber The initial interest focussed on the effects of fiber in modifying carbohydrate and lipid metabolism. The slower rate of absorption was not however associated with gross carbohydrate malabsorption as judged by breath H_2[20] and urinary xylose excretion[21] studies. Nevertheless the viscous types of fiber, which showed the greatest metabolic effects on glucose and lipid metabolism were also those which were degraded by the colonic microflora. The products of bacterial fermentation of fiber include the short chain volatile fatty acids acetate, propionate and butyrate which are largely absorbed from the colon.[22] In ruminants propionate induces satiety and enhances insulin secretion.[23] In man the closely related ketoacids acetoacetate and 3-OH butyrate have been shown to suppress FFA release (Fig 4)[24] and in the presence of carbohydrate to enhance insulin secretion.[25]

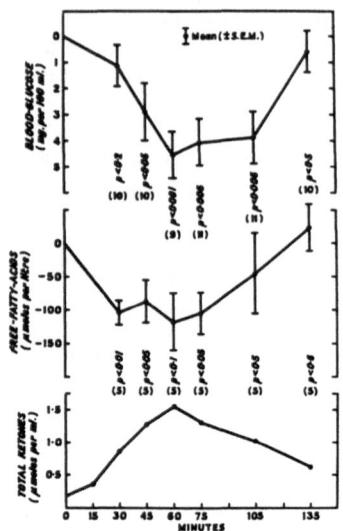

FIGURE 4. Changes in blood glucose and plasma F.F.A. from initial levels shown as means of differences between test (acetoacetate) and control (saline solution) experiments, and total blood-ketone bodies (mean of two test experiments).[24]

It is thus possible that some of the chronic effects of fiber on carbohydrate and lipid metabolism may relate to the absorbed products of colonic degradation of fiber. For example induction of reduced FFA levels would favour increased insulin binding of hepatocytes and thus favour a reduction in net glucose output by the liver.[26] In this way the basal glucose levels would be influenced by the chronic effects of fiber and the acute effects would be reflected in reduced post prandial glucose levels.

Because of the combined experience with high fiber diets and the physiological implications of increased fiber consumption, high fiber diets were advocated such that glycemic control could be maintained or improved while the carbohydrate content of the diet was raised. This has formed the rationale for the higher fiber, higher carbohydrate diets currently recommended.

2.2 Glycemic response to starchy foods

It is now recognised that the differences in glycemic response to different starchy foods is related to many characteristics of foods and not simply to their dietary fiber content.[27,28] Thus white bread and spaghetti are similar in terms of their chemical composition but spaghetti produces a much flatter glycemic response than does bread [29] (Fig 5).

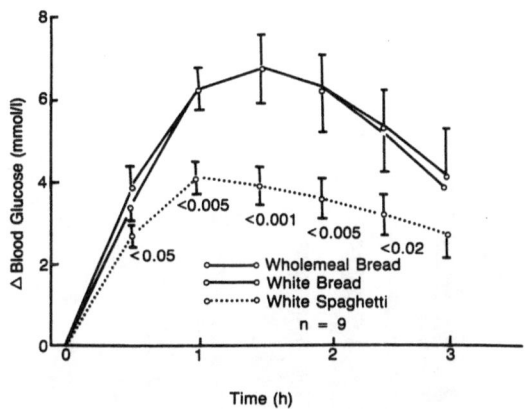

FIGURE 5. Mean blood glucose increments after equicarbohydrate meals of wholemeal and white breads and spaghetti given to diabetic volunteers. P values are given for the difference between the mean of the bread meals and spaghetti.[29]

Classification of foods in terms of their glycemic effect by comparison with a reference food (eg white bread) allows selection of those foods which for a given amount of carbohydrate raise the blood glucose the least. Up until now only a limited number of foods have been classified according to their glycemic indices, however there is general agreement between values established in non-diabetic individuals and patients with both insulin dependent (IDDM) and non-insulin dependent diabetes (NIDDM) [27] Greater variability in the IDDM patients in terms of fasting blood glucose levels and glucose tolerance status also means that the GI values established for IDDM have greater coefficients of variation.

In the future, recommendations may be based on the actual glycemic effect[30-35] of foods (glycemic index) but at present, too few foods have been tested to make this practical in the standard clinical setting (Fig 6).

2.3 Fiber, Lente Carbohyrate and Trials of Diabetic Therapy

The majority of successful trials of fiber supplements or high fiber foods used in the treatment of diabetics have involved the use of fibers which impede carbohydrate absorption[15,36-38] or of high fiber foods[39-43] (especially legumes) with a slow rate of in vitro digestion [44](Fig 7).

Although the studies were not specifically designed to test the effects of incorporation of sustained release or lente carbohydrate into the diabetic diet, their success indicates the potential usefulness of this approach. No studies have been undertaken where the effects of differences in the nature of the available carbohydrate have been examined separately from fiber content. The long term benefits of specifically reducing the post prandial glycemia remain to be assessed. However studies where the glycemic response has been reduced by

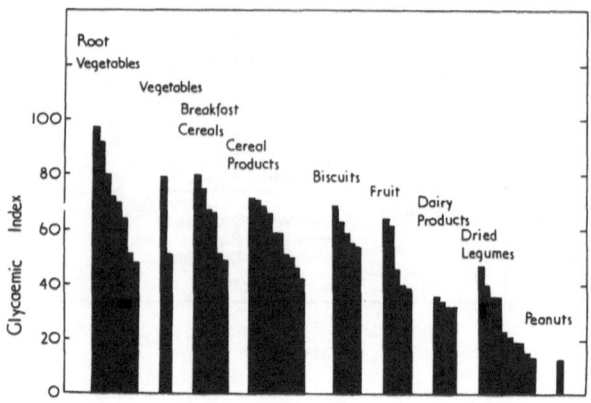

FIGURE 6. Glycemic index of foods (i.e. incremental area under the 2h blood glucose curve of 50g carbohydrate food portions, 50g glucose itself being 100%). Each bar in each block represents the mean result for one food tested by 5-10 individuals.[30]

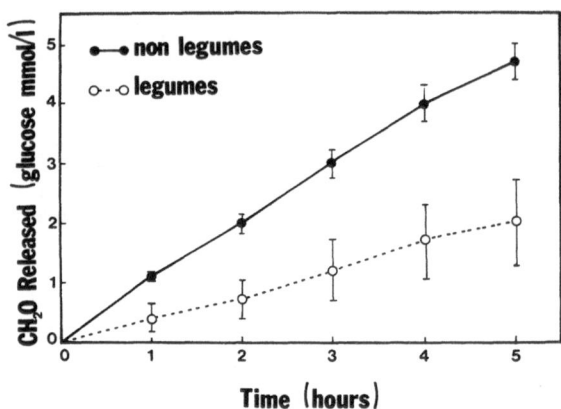

Time (hours)

FIGURE 7. The increase in concentration over 5h of the products of starch digestion, measured as glucose after acid hydrolysis, subsequent to incubation of 2g available carbohydrate portions of foods with pooled human saliva and pancreatic juice. For legumes (e.g. red lentils and kidney beans) and non-legumes (e.g. wholemeal bread, instant mashed potato, rice, spaghetti and millet).[44]

α-glycoside hydrolase inhibition[45,46] have indicated improvement in diabetic control. In addition it is of interest that the second meal carbohydrate tolerance is improved in normal volunteers following a low glycemic index food taken as the preceding meal.[47]

3. CARBOHYDRATE INTAKE AND BLOOD LIPIDS

Since a reduction in blood lipids, notably cholesterol, has been one of the reasons for the advice given to reduce fat intake it is important that the carbohydrates used do not raise the other major serum lipid component, triglyceride. Some of the reasons for this concern stem from studies of high carbohydrate formula diets fed to poorly controlled diabetics[48] and 10 day metabolic studies using common foods in normal volunteers.[49] There is also evidence that certain sugars (fructose and sucrose) in specific situations,[50-53] though not in others[54-55] may result in raised blood lipids. However studies where the carbohydrate intake has been increased using high fiber starchy foods (such as legumes) have actually resulted in reductions in serum cholesterol and also serum triglyceride.[56-58] Most recently use of increased amounts of low glycemic index starchy foods with relatively small changes in total fiber intake have been shown to lower total and LDL cholesterol and serum triglyceride levels in hyperlipidemic volunteers [59] (Fig 8). Thus both food components such as fiber and the physiological characteristics of the starch are likely to influence serum lipids and provide new approaches to the dietary therapy not only of diabetes but also of hyperlipidemia.

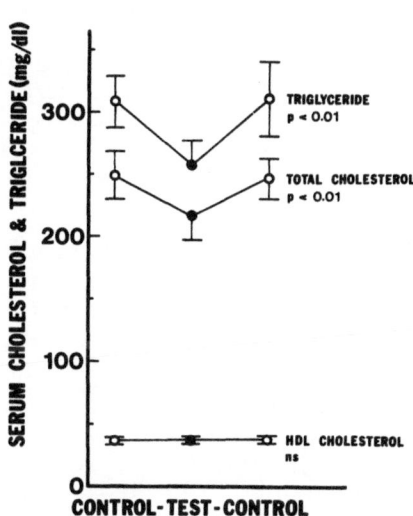

FIGURE 8. Mean total serum cholesterol, triglyceride and HDL cholesterol levels (10 patients) during a 3 month study during the middle month of which low glycemic index foods were substituted into the diet without altering the fiber or macronutrient composition. The values represent the mean of the fasting samples taken at the end of the second and fourth week of each month.[59]

4. DIETARY PROTEIN

Attention has been drawn to the use of increased protein in the diabetic diet to reduce the fat and carbohydrate content. However, many animal protein foods also tend to be high in saturated fat. Perhaps of even greater concern is the effect of increased nitrogen metabolism on renal function. This is especially so in view of the current research indicating that renal function can be preserved by early reduction in protein intake,[60-61] a matter of obvious relevance to the treatment of diabetics. It therefore seems unlikely that high protein intakes will ever be adopted as part of the dietary treatment of diabetics.

5. CONCLUSION

Current dietary advice in the management of diabetes has emphasized a reduction in fat intake and an increase in the intake of carbohydrate foods especially those rich in dietary fibre. Attention has been drawn to the differences in physiological response to different carbohydrate foods and the need for classification on the basis of their glycemic effect. Studies have indicated that use of appropriate foods may benefit both blood glucose control and reduce blood lipids. Pharmacological offshoots of this approach in terms of fibre supplements (or supplemented foods) and enzyme inhibitors are also undergoing development.

REFERENCES

(1) Stone DB, Connor WE. Prolonged effects of a low cholesterol, high carbohydrate diet upon the serum lipids in diabetic patients. Diabetes 1965;12:127-132.

(2) Weinsier RL, Seeman A, Henera MG, Assal JP, Soeldner JS, Gleason RE. High and low carbohydrate diets in diabetes mellitus. Study of effects on diabetic control. Insulin secretion and blood lipids. Ann Intern Med 1974;80:332-341.

(3) Brunzell JD, Lerner RL, Hazard WR, Porte D, Bierman EL. Improved glucose tolerance with high carbohydrate feeding in mild diabetes. New Eng J Med 1971;284:521-524.

(4) Dayton S, Pearce ML, Goldman H, Harnish A, Plotkin D, Shickman M, Winfield M, Zager A, Dixon W. Controlled trial of a diet high in unsaturated fat for prevention of atherosclerotic complications. Lancet 1968; 2:1060-1062.

(5) Miettinen T, Turpeinen O, Karvonen MN, Elosuo K, Poavilainen E. Effect of cholesterol-lowering diet on mortality from coronary heart disease and other causes: a twelve year clinical trial in men and women. Lancet 1972; 2:835-838.

(6) The Lipid Research Clinics Coronary Primary Prevention Trial Results: 1: Reduction in incidence of coronary heart disease JAMA 1984; 251:351-64.

(7) Committee of the American Diabetes Association on Food and Nutrition Special Report: Principles of nutrition and dietary recommendtions for individuals with diabetes mellitus. Diabetes Care 1979; 2:520-523.

(8) Special Report Committee Guidelines for the nutritional management of diabetes mellitus: A special report from the Canadian Diabetes Association. J Can Dietet Assoc 1981; 42:110-118.

(9) The Nutrition Sub-Committee of the British Diabetic Association's Medical Advisory Committee: Dietary recommendations for diabetes for the 1980's - A policy statement by the British Diabetic Association. Human Nutr: Applied Nutr 1982; 36A:378-394.

(10) Report of the Ad Hoc Committee on Glycemic Effects of Carbohydrates. Council on Nutrition, American Diabetes Association February 1984.

(11) Jenkins DJA, Leeds AR, Gassull MA, Wolever TMS, Goff DV, Alberti KGMM, Hockaday TDR. Unabsorbble carbohydrates and diabetes: decreased post prandial hyperglycaemia. Lancet 1976;2:172-174.

(12) Jenkins DJA, Wolever TMS, Hockaday TDR, Leeds AR, Haworth R, Bacon S, Apling EC, Dilawari J. Treatment of diabetes with guar gum. Lancet 1977;2:779-780.

(13) Jenkins DJA, Wolver TMS, Nineham R, Goff DV, Haisman P, Charnock P, Taylor RH, Hockaday TDR. Dietary fibre and ketone bodies: reduced urinary 3-hydroxybutyrate excretion in diabetics on guar. Brit Med J 1979;2:1555-1556.

(14) Jenkins DJA, Wolever TMS, Taylor, Reynolds D, Nineham R, Hockaday TDR. Diabetic glucose control, lipids, and trace elements on long term guar. Brit Med J 1980;1:1353-1354.

(15) Aro A, Uusitupa M, Vontilainen E, Hersio K, Korhonen T, Siitonen O. Improved diabetic control and hypocholesterolemic effect induced by long term dietary supplementation with guar gum in type 2 (insulin-independent) diabetes. Diabetologia 1981;21:29-33.

(16) Smith U, Holm. G. Effect of a modified guar gum preparation on glucose and lipid levels in diabetics and healthy volunteers. Atherosclerosis 1982;45:1-10.

(17) Anderson JW, Ward K. Long-term effects of high carbohydrate, high fiber diets on glucose and lipid metabolism: A preliminary report on patients with diabetes. Diabetes Care 1978;1:77-82.

(18) Anderson JW, Chen WL. Plant fiber: Carbohydrate and lipid metabolism. Am J Clin Nutr 1979;32:346-363.

(19) Anderson JW, Ward K. High carbohydrate, high fiber diets for insulin treated men with diabetes mellitus. Am J Clin Nutr 1979;32:2312-2321.

(20) Jenkins DJA, Leeds AR, Gassull MA, Cochet B, Alberti KGMM. Decrease in postprandial insulin and glucose concentrations by guar and pectin. Ann Int Med 1977;86:20-23.

(21) Jenkins DJA, Wolever TMS, Leeds AR, Gassull MA, Dilawari JB, Goff DV, Metz GL, Alberti KGMM. Dietary fibres, fibre analogues and glucose tolerance: importance of viscosity. Brit Med J 1978;1:1392-1394.

(22) Cummings JH. Short chain fatty acids in the human colon. Gut 1981;22:763-779.

(23) Istasse L, Goodall EO, Orskov ER. The effect of ruminal infusions of propionic acid or abomasal infusion of glucose on plasma insulin secretion in non-lactating cows. Proc Nutr Soc 1984;44:45A.

(24) Jenkins DJA. Ketone bodies and the inhibition of free-fatty-acid release. Lancet 1967;2:338-40.

(25) Jenkins DJA, Hunter WM, Goff DV. Ketone bodies and evidence for increased insulin secretion. Nature 1970;227:384-5.

(26) Bjorntorp P, Sjostrom L. Adipose tissue dysfunction and its consequences. In: Cryer, A, Van K. Eds. New perspective in adipose tissue. London Butterworth 1984.

(27) Jenkins DJA, Wolever TMS, Jenkins AL, Josse RG, Wong GS. The glycaemic response to carbohydrate foods. Lancet 1984;2:388-391.

(28) Crapo PA, Insel J, Sperling M, Kolterman OG. Comparison of serum glucose, insulin, and glucagon responses to different types of complex carbohydrate in non-insulin dependent diabetic patients. Am J Clin Nutr 1981;34:184-190.

(29) Jenkins DJA, Wolever TMS, Jenkins AL, Lee R, Wong GS, Josse R. Glycemic response to wheat products: reduced response to pasta but no effect of fiber. Diabetes Care 1983;6:155-159.

(30) Jenkins DJA, Wolever TMS, Taylor RH, Barker H, Fielden H, Baldwin JM, Bowling AC, Newman HC, Jenkins AL, Goff DV. Glycemic index of foods: A physiological basis for carbohydrate exchange. Am J Clin Nutr 1981; 34:362-366.

(31) Jenkins DJA, Wolever TMS. Slow release carbohydrate and the treatment of diabetes. Proc Nutr Soc 1981;40:227-235.

(32) Jenkins DJA, Wolever TMS, Jenkins AL, Thorne MJ, Lee K, Kalmusky J, Reichert R, Wong GS. The glycemic index of foods tested in diabetic patients: A new basis for carbohydrate exchange favouring the use of legumes. Diabetologia 1983; 24:257-264.

(33) Schauberger G, Brinck UC, Guldner G, Spaethe R, Niklas L, Otto H. Exchange of carbohydrates according to their effect on blood glucose. Diabetes 1977; 26:415.

(34) Crapo PA, Reaven G, Olefsky J. Plasma glucose and insulin responses to orally administered simple and complex carbohydrates. Diabetes 1976; 25:741-747.

(35) Crapo PA, Reaven GM, Olefsky J. Post-prandial plasma glucose responses to different complex carbohydrates. Diabetes 1977; 26:1178-83.

(36) Jenkins DJA, Wolever TMS, Bacon S, Nineham R, Leeds R, Rowden R, Love M, Hockaday TDR. Diabetic diets: high carbohydrate combined with high fibre. Am J Clin Nutr 1980; 33:1729-1733.

(37) Jenkins DJA, Wolever TMS, Nineham R, Taylor R, Metz GL, Bacon S, Hockaday TDR. Guar crispbread in the diabetic diet. Br Med J 1978; 2:1744-1746.

(38) Doi K, Matsuura M, Kawasa A, Baba S. Treatment of diabetes with glucomannan (Konjac mannan). Lancet 1979; 1:987-988.

(39) Anderson JW, Ward K. Long-term effects of high carbohydrate, high fiber diets on glucose and lipid metabolism. A preliminary report on patients with diabetes. Diabetes Care 1978; 1:77-82.

(40) Anderson JW, Chen WL. Plant fiber carbohydrate and lipid metabolism. Am J Clin Nutr 1979; 32:346-363.

(41) Anderson JW, Ward K. High carbohydrate high fiber diets for insulin-treated men with diabetes mellitus. Am J Clin Nutr 1979; 32:2312-2321.

(42) Simpson HCR, Simpson RW, Lousley S, Carter RD, Geekie M, Hockaday TDR, Mann JI. A high carbohydrate leguminous fibre diet improves all aspects of diabetic control. Lancet 1981; 1:1-5.

(43) Rivellese A, Riccardi G, Giacco A, Pacioni D, Genovese S, Mattioli PL, Mancini M. Effect of dietary fibre on glucose control and serum lipoproteins in diabetic patients. Lancet 1980; 2:447-450.

(44) Jenkins DJA, Ghafari H, Wolever TMS, Taylor RH, Barker HM, Fielden H, Jenkins AL, Bowling AC. Relationship between the rate of digestion of foods and post-prandial glycaemia. Diabetologia 1982; 22:6.

(45) Lambert AE, Damoiseaux P, Buysschaert M, Hillebrand I, Kelelslegers JM. Improved glycemic control in type I diabetes. In First International Symposium on Acarbose. Ed W. Creutzfeldt. Excerpta Medica. Oxford 1982; pp 417-21.

(46) Walton RJ, Sherif IT, Noy GA, Albert KGMM. Improved metabolic profiles in insulin-treated diabetic patients given an alpha-glucoside hydrolase inhibitor. Br Med J 1979; 1:220-1.

(47) Jenkins DJA, Wolever TMS, Taylor RH, Griffiths C, Krzeminska K, Lawrie JA, Bennett CM, Goff DV, Sarson DL, Bloom SR. Slow release carbohydrate improves second meal tolerance. Am J Clin Nutr 1982; 35:1339-1346.

(48) Brunzell JD, Lerner RI, Porte D, Bierman EL. Effect of a fat free, high carbohydrate diet on diabetic subjects with fasting hyperglycemia. Diabetes 1979; 23:138-142.

(49) Coulston AM, Liu GC, Reaven GM. Plasma glucose, insulin and lipid responses to high carbohydrate low fat diets in normal humans. Metabolism 1983; 32:52-56.

(50) Kuo PT, Bassett DR. Dietary Sugar in the production of hypertriglyceridemia. Ann Int. Med 1965; 62:1199.

(51) Reiser S, Hallfrisch J, Michaelis O, Lagar FL, Martin RE, Prather ES. Isocaloric exchange of dietary starch and sucrose in humans: Effects on levels of fasting blood lipids. Am J Clin Nutr 1978; 32:1659-1669.

(52) Antar MA, Little JA, Lucas C, Buckley GC, Csima A. Interrelationships between the kinds of dietary carbohydrate and fat in hyperlipoproteinemic patients. Part 3. Synergistic effect of sucrose and animal fat on serum lipids. Atherosclerosis 1970; 11:191-201.

(53) MacDonald I, Braithwaite DM. The influence of dietary carbohydrates on the lipid pattern in serum and adipose tissue. Clin Sci 1964; 27:23.

(54) Grande F, Anderson JT, Keys A. Sucrose and various carbohydrate containing foods and serum lipids in man. Am J Clin Nutr 1974; 27:1043-1051.

(55) Turner JL, Bierman EL, Brunzell JD, Chart A. Effect of dietary fructose on triglyceride transport and glucoregulatory hormones in hypertriglyceridemic men. Am J Clin Nutr 1979; 32:1043-50.

(56) Anderson JW. High carbohydrate, high fiber diets for patients with diabetes. In: Camerini-Davalos RA, Hanover BA (eds). Treatment of Early Diabetes. Plenum Press, New York, 1979; pp 263-273.

(57) Simpson RW, Mann JI, Eaton J, Moore RA, Carter R, Hockaday TDR. Improved glucose control in maturity onset diabetes treated with carbohydrate-modified fat diet. Br Med J 1979; 1:1752-1756.

(58) Jenkins DJA, Wong GS, Patten R, Bird J, Hall M, Buckley GC, McGuire V, Reichert R, Little JA. Leguminous seeds in the dietary management of hyperlipidemia. Am J Clin Nutr 1983; 38:567-573.

(59) Jenkins DJA, Wolever TMS, Kalmusky J, Guidici S, Giordano C, Wong GS, Bird JN, Patten R, Hall M, Buckley G, Little JA. Low glycemic index foods in the management of hyperlipidemia. Am J Clin Nutr 1985 in Press.

(60) EL Nahas AM, Masters-Thomas A, Brady SA, Famington K, Wilkinson V, Hilson AJW, Varghese Z, Moorhead JF. Selective low protein diets in chronic renal diseases. Brit Med J 1984; 298:1337-1341.

(61) Rosman JB, Ter Wee PM, Meiger S, Piers-Becht TPLM, Sluiter WJ, Donker AJM. Prospective randomized trial of early dietary protein restriction in chronic renal failure. Lancet 1984; 2:1291-1296.

2.1.3. Oral hypoglycaemic drugs
H. Keen and S. Ng Tang Fui

1. INTRODUCTION
    Oral hypoglycaemic agents, principally the sulphonylureas
are today widely used in the treatment of patients with
non-insulin dependent diabetes mellitus (NIDDM) who make up
75-80% of the total diabetic population. The rationale for
their use includes both the short term aims of relief of
symptoms and biochemical correction and the longer term
aspiration for protection against the long-term
complications of the diabetic state, affecting eyes,
kidneys, nerves and arteries. The short-term aims are
certainly achievable, at least in the short run, but there
is conflicting and incomplete evidence as to their
preventive efficacy for diabetic complications. The advent
of the oral agents has certainly not eradicated them.
    While the number of sulphonylurea derivatives introduced
into therapy continues to multiply there remain areas of
uncertainty in the understanding of their mode of action.
Other orally active preparations, notably the biguanides but
also a number of novel compounds, have also been
investigated, to a greater or lesser extent, and brief
reference will be made to these in the selective review
which follows. The optimistic and uncritical use of oral
agents for the decade or so after their introduction has
given place to the realisation that they are no magic
'monotherapy' for diabetes and that adequate management must
include concern with diet and with the correction of other
risk factors (e.g. hypertension, hyperlipidaemia, cigarette
smoking) which play an important part in determining
outcome. The oral agents represent a useful part, but only
part of the management of diabetes 'on a broad front'.

2. HISTORICAL ASPECTS
    The first substantial pharmaceutical approach to the
treatment of diabetes with oral agents was with aspirin,
more than a century ago (1). The prime concern then was to
find some therapy for the otherwise lethal insulin-dependent
variety of the disease (IDDM). The guanidine derivatives,
synthalin A and B provoked some interest as oral
antidiabetic agents in the early 1920's (2) but were
moderately toxic and in any case were eclipsed by the advent
of insulin which provided an effective answer to the most
pressing problems of IDDM. It was a chance discovery during
World War II in France by Janbon, confirmed experimentally
by Loubatieres (3), of the hypoglycaemic properties of a
sulphonamide derivative being investigated for its

antibacterial activity in typhoid fever, that rekindled
interest in oral antidiabetic agents. It was not until the
1950's that Franke and Fuchs (4) further exploited these
wartime observations and opened the current era of oral
hypoglycaemic agents with the systematic study of the
sulphonylureas. At about the same time, revived interest in
the guanidine derivatives gave rise to the biguanides (5) as
a second class of oral antidiabetic agents.

Carbutamide , the first widely used sulphonylurea (4),
was withdrawn after comparatively few years of trial due to
bone marrow toxicity. Soon after, tolbutamide (6) and
chlorpropamide (7) became established as effective
hypoglycaemic sulphonylureas and were widely introduced into
the treatment of NIDDM. It was recognised very early that
they were effective only in patients with adequate
endogenous insulin secretory capacity and totally
ineffective in patients with IDDM. The few diabetics in
whom they appeared to replace insulin injections were those
NIDDM patients being so treated because of failure to
respond to diet. Sustained ketonuria at onset virtually
excluded successful use of oral agents and they were
ineffective even in some non-ketonuric diabetics (primary
failure).

The 1960's saw the expanding and uncritical use of the
oral agents in NIDDM. In addition to their use in
clinically manifest patients, the discovery of large numbers
of asymptomatic mildly hyperglycaemic individuals in
population surveys introduced a preventive dimension in
their application, the hope that they might delay metabolic
deterioration in people with 'early', 'borderline' or
'chemical' diabetes (8).

3. EPIDEMIOLOGY OF ANTIDIABETIC THERAPY

The use of oral hypoglycaemic agents varies considerably
from population to population. Table I shows the proportion
of diabetic patients recruited to the WHO Multinational
Study (9) who were receiving the three main forms of
treatment: diet alone, oral hypoglycaemic drugs and insulin.
Each centre participating in this study introduced
approximately 500 patients, aged 35-55 years and stratified
to provide similar known durations of diabetes. The wide
variation in the proportion in this age-group receiving
oral agents reflects the relative frequency of
insulin-dependent patients in these populations as well as
prevailing local therapeutic practices. In the mid 1970's,
almost 2% of the population of Germany were taking oral
antidiabetic preparations (10) and Wade (11) has shown great
variation in the use of oral agents within part of the UK.

Some of the variation in use of oral agents is related to
the impact of the results of the US University Group
Diabetes Programme (UGDP) study of the early 1970's (12).
In this multicentre trial, newly diagnosed NIDDM patients
were all recommended a diet, then randomly assigned to
treatment with placebo tablets, tolbutamide (1.5g/day),
insulin at a fixed or at a variable dose level or, in an

TABLE I: TREATMENT PATTERNS IN WHO MULTINATIONAL STUDY

	INSULIN	ORAL DRUGS	DIET ONLY
London	58.8 %	29.4 %	11.8%
Switzerland	56.2	35.3	8.6
Brussels	51.2	25.7	23.7
Moscow	46.3	40.4	13.3
Warsaw	59.5	35.0	5.5
Berlin (GDR)	46.4	28.2	25.5
Zagreb	36.9	41.1	21.9
New Delhi	22.7	67.2	10.2
Hong Kong	34.0	64.4	1.7
Tokyo	31.5	46.2	22.8
Havana	26.6	59.8	13.6
Oklahoma	21.3	52.1	26.7
Arizona	33.7	28.7	37.7
Bulgaria	51.8	41.2	7.1
TOTAL (n=6695)	41.0	43.2	15.6
MEN (n=3301)	41.5	42.0	16.5
WOMEN (n=3394)	40.5	44.4	15.2

Proportions of the age (35-54), sex, diabetes duration
stratified national diabetic samples recruited receiving
treatment with insulin, oral drugs or diet only.
N.B. Both U.S samples were of Amerindian diabetics.

extension of the study, to phenformin, 100mg/day. The aim
was to compare the efficacy of these treatments in
controlling glycaemia and reducing diabetic complications.
After about 6 years an apparent excess of cardiovascular and
sudden death appeared to be emerging in the
tolbutamide-treated group compared with the placebo group
and the sulphonylurea was therefore discontinued. It is
noteworthy that in this rigorously debated and criticised
trial, coronary mortality was unexpectedly low in the
placebo treated group, none of its 21 deaths being assigned
to coronary cause (13). Although four other randomly
allocated, double blind trials of tolbutamide versus placebo
(14-17) offered no support for this disconcerting finding,
there nevertheless followed a considerable decline in
sulphonylurea usage in the US.
    Oral agents reached their apogee with the withdrawal of
phenformin. This was not so much because of the further
UGDP report of increased cardiovascular mortality as to the
growing evidence that the use of the drug in diabetes led to
an increased risk of lactic acidosis (18).

3.1 Cardiac effects of tolbutamide
    The main doubts raised by the UGDP reports concerned the
possible adverse cardiovascular effects of tolbutamide.
This led to a number of laboratory and clinical studies of
the effect of the drug on cardiac activity. Several

investigations in animals suggested some positive inotropic
effect but there were clear species differences (19).
Studies in man were limited and contradictory (20,21). As
part of an investigation of insulin release and glycaemic
response to sulphonylureas, we incorporated a study of the
acute effects of intravenous bolus doses of tolbutamide on
systolic time intervals . In 7 normal volunteers, 7 IDDM
and 7 NIDDM patients aged 42-63 years, we made simultaneous
recordings of electrocardiograms, phonocardiograms and
carotid pulse wave traces, at rest and for 45 mins following
each of two intravenous bolus doses of sodium tolbutamide
(50 and 250 mg). For positive control purposes, the study

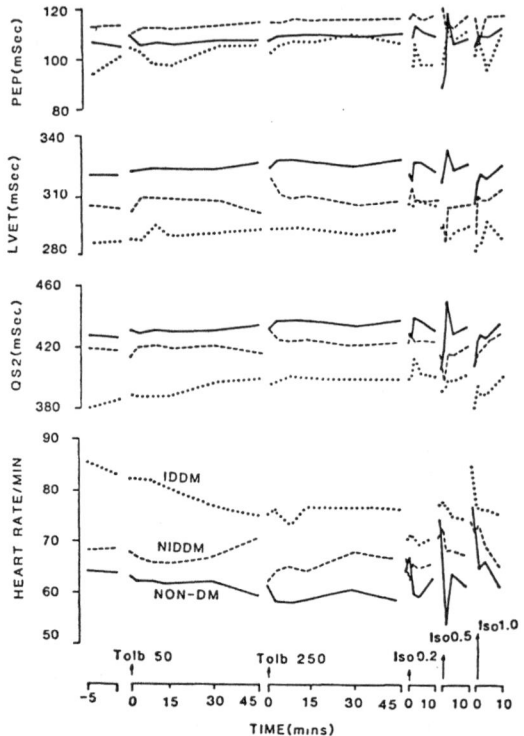

FIG 1: The effect of 2 iv boluses of tolbutamide 50 and 250mg respectively
on heart rate and systolic time intervals (QS$_2$, LVET and PEP corrected for
heart rate) in 7 non-diabetics, 7 IDDM and 7 NIDDM volunteers. QS$_2$(interval
between Q wave and 2nd heart sound) represents total electromechanical
systolic time. LVET= left ventricular ejection time, measured as carotid
upstroke to incisura. PEP (pre-ejection period) is the duration of
electrical activation and isometric contraction of left ventricle=QS$_2$-LVET.
   Following basal observations, recordings were made for 45mins after
each tolbutamide bolus dose, followed by a 'washout'period of 30mins.
3 isoprenaline (ISO) boluses of 0.2, 0.5 and 1.0ug respectively were then
given with 10mins recording for each, followed by 10mins 'washout' interval
No significant inotropic or chronotropic effects followed tolbutamide
compared to isoprenaline.

was completed with observations on the effects of three small bolus doses of isoprenaline (0.2, 0.5 and 1.0 ug). The systolic time intervals QS_2, PEP and LVET as defined in Fig 1 were calculated. No significant chronotropic or inotropic effects of tolbutamide could be found (Fig 1) though even for the smallest isoprenaline dose clear effects were recorded. While these experiments do not exclude a long-term cardiac effect of tolbutamide, it gives no support to the view that the drug has a significant direct inotropic effect in man. Two of the treated NIDDM patients had in fact previously been receiving long term tolbutamide therapy and did not differ in their responses from the rest of the subjects.

3.2 THE UK PROSPECTIVE STUDY

The residual conflict of evidence over the sulphonylureas may be resolved by the Multicentre UK Prospective Study of Therapies of Maturity-Onset Diabetes (22), now in its fifth year. This study involving 15 clinical centres and aiming to recruit some 3,500 newly diagnosed NIDDM patients, bears only superficial resemblance to UGDP and has a more clinically realistic (and complex) design. Essentially, patients aged 25-65 years recruited to the trial are initially treated with diet only for 3 months. If they fail to achieve a fasting blood glucose value below 7 mmol/L and are not obese, they are randomly allocated to treatment either with continued diet alone (30%), to insulin treatment (30%), to chlorpropamide (20%) or to glibenclamide (20%). For patients over 20% above ideal weight, a metformin treatment option is added. Treatment response is optimised with an agreed adjustable dosage scale. If oral agents fail, patients are changed to insulin. In an early report (22) 777 patients had been recruited and 286 followed for one year. The glycaemic response to oral agents was comparable to ultralente insulin and clearly superior to diet alone. A high proportion of those responding initially to diet alone failed to maintain the response over the following year and were randomised to one of the treatment groups. The treatment goals of this study are based upon the therapeutic philosophy (23) that, if the setting level of the overnight fasting plasma glucose can be adequately lowered, the glycaemic profile for the whole day will follow suit.

The UK Prospective Study asks a number of clinically important questions. Can adequate glycaemic control be achieved equally well in NIDDM with oral agents and insulin? Will improved control protect the patient from complications? Are there advantages for either insulin or oral agents from the point of view of efficacy, acceptability, and protection from complications? Peacock and Tattersall (24) considered the problem of the use of insulin in NIDDM patients with suboptimal control on oral agents alone. In a crossover comparison between insulin (Monotard once daily to a maximum of 48 units) and oral agents (glibenclamide up to 20mg/day with metformin up to 2g daily) they were unable to show mean glycaemic advantage of one treatment over the other. However, in a third of their patients, control was better on insulin (unchanged in a third and worse in a third). They concluded that only by trial can potential improvement with their simple insulin regime be demonstrated and that in a substantial number of patients, responses may be as good or better on oral agents. This conclusion can only be applied to the simple and dose-limited insulin regimen they used.

4. SULPHONYLUREAS

At least 10 sulphonylurea preparations are now available (Table II). The common sulphonylurea core determines hypoglycaemic activity and the different terminal substituents account for differences in pharmacological properties and potency. The more recently introduced agents are sometimes known as 'second generation' sulphonylureas to distinguish them from the earlier compounds but, apart from their general property of lower .dose requirement (Table II), there are no major differences in their pharmacological actions or efficacy.

TABLE II: ORAL HYPOGLYCAEMIC DRUGS

SULPHONYLUREAS R_1-⟨⟩-SO_2-NH-CO-NH-R_2		TOTAL DAILY DOSE(mg)	DOSES PER DAY	PLASMA HALF LIFE(h)	DURATION HYPOGLY EFFECT(h)	METABOLISM	URINE EXCRE- TION %
ACETOHEXAMIDE	Dimelor	250–1000	2–3	7 ± 1	15 ± 3	H reduct*	60
CHLORPROPAMIDE	Diabenese, Melitase	100–500	1	36	60	H hydrox*	90
GLIBENCLAMIDE	Daonil, Euglucon	2.5–20	1–2	8 ± 4	18 ± 6	H	50
GLIBORNURIDE	Glutril	12.5–75	1–2	8	18 ± 6	H	65
GLICLAZIDE	Diamicron	80–320	1–2	12	12	H	
GLIPIZIDE	Glibenese, Minodiab	2.5–30	2–3	8	18 ± 6	H	70
GLIQUIDONE	Glurenorm	15–180	3	2	4	H	**
GLYMIDINE	Gondafon	500–2000	1–3	6 ± 2	8 ± 2	H*	
TOLAZAMIDE	Tolanase	100–1000	1–2	7	12	H	85
TOLBUTAMIDE	Rastinon, Pramidex	500–3000	2–3	5	9 ± 3	H carbox	100
BIGUANIDES $\underset{R_2}{\overset{R_1}{>}}$N-C-NH-C-NH$_2$ (H, H)							
METFORMIN	Glucophage	500–3000	1–3		18 ± 6		100

H=Hepatic. * Metabolites active. ** Excreted via liver and/or kidney. R_1 & R_2 represent substituent sites.

4.1 Mode of Action

There are two mechanisms by which sulphonylureas are thought to reduce hyperglycaemia in NIDDM (Fig 2): (1) by augmenting insulin secretion from the B-cells of the pancreatic islets (a central or pancreatic effect), (2) by enhancing the action of circulating insulin on target tissues (peripheral or extrapancreatic effects). The extrapancreatic effects could occur in the liver and/or in peripheral tissues such as adipose tissue and muscle. It is generally accepted that sulphonylureas directly increase insulin secretion in the early stages of therapy (25). However it has been questioned whether this direct mechanism is still important after the first few weeks or months of treatment (indeed whether a pancreatic effect is present at all) or whether the major locus of action is extrapancreatic (26-28).

FIG 2: MODE OF ACTION OF SULPHONYLUREAS

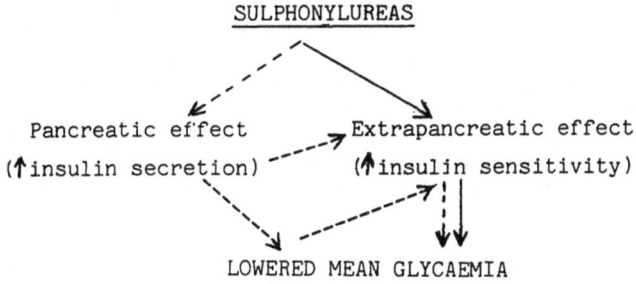

4.1.1. Pancreatic effect of sulphonylureas: The pancreatic action of sulphonylureas has been recognised since the early observations of Loubatieres (3) who demonstrated the release of an insulin-like substance from the pancreas of experimental animals. There was no effect in pancreatectomised (29) or alloxan-induced (30) diabetic animals. Later studies (31) confirmed that short term administration of sulphonylureas to NIDDM patients produced an increase in plasma insulin concentration, associated with a fall in plasma glucose. These observations and the lack of sulphonylurea effect in insulin-dependent patients without endogenous insulin secretory capacity (32) strongly suggested that sulphonylureas act in NIDDM patients by increasing insulin secretion.

The mechanism of the insulin release response is still under investigation. There is evidence that sulphonylureas stimulate insulin secretion without penetrating the B-cell (33) suggesting a primary effect through interaction with structures on the B-cell plasma membrane. Recent studies (34,35) suggest that insulin release is triggered by intracellular calcium ion redistribution, either directly (through increases in calcium efflux) or indirectly, secondary to changes in transmembrane fluxes of potassium or sodium ions. Sulphonylureas stimulate the acute release of preformed insulin but do not accelerate insulin synthesis (33). They also reduce depolarisation of the B-cell membrane, increase electrical activity of the cell and reduce transmembrane potassium flux (36). Ashcroft et al (37) have presented interesting new evidence on the association of glucose-induced increased electrical activity of the B-cell, its depolarisation and diminished cell membrane permeability to potassium ions. This appears to be linked with the closure of a specific potassium channel (G channel), apparently controlled by ambient glucose concentration. This G channel might be influenced by sulphonylureas and other insulin secretagogues. The earlier suggestion of Loubatieres (3) of stimulation of formation of new B-cells by sulphonylureas has not been substantiated (38).

In studies with 18 NIDDM patients, Judzewitsch et al (39) have constructed 'dose-response' curves of the acute islet insulin secretory response to a fixed arginine stimulus at three plasma glucose levels before and during chlorpropamide therapy. When the pre-therapy fasting plasma glucose was matched by glucose infusion during chlorpropamide treatment, the acute insulin response was considerably increased. They concluded that chlorpropamide restores a more nearly normal islet responsiveness to glucose.

4.1.2. Extrapancreatic effects of sulphonylureas: The notion that sulphonylurea effects might not be solely attributable to B-cell stimulation and increased insulin secretion was based on two observations. Firstly, after some weeks of successful sulphonylurea therapy in NIDDM, although blood glucose levels remained low, elevation of plasma insulin levels was no longer demonstrated (40). Secondly, in a substantial number of responsive patients therapy could be withdrawn after an interval with persisting improvement of glycaemic control (41).These findings, suggesting some extrapancreatic change which enhances the effectiveness of (reduces resistance to) the action of insulin are not at issue. What is less certain is their mechanism (Fig 2). Is it due to a direct effect of the sulphonylurea on non B-cell tissues? Is it a protracted tissue response to the initial increase in insulin secretion? Or is it the tissue consequence of a period of improved glycaemic control, however achieved? These questions might be answered by a clearer understanding of how the 'improved' tissue response is generated. Is it due to humoral or hormonal changes, to effects on membrane receptors for insulin or to modifications in the post receptor events which mediate the intracellular actions of insulin? A further set of questions is directed to the anatomical site of the extrapancreatic effects; is glycaemia reduced by restraint upon hepatic glucose output, by increased utilisation of glucose by peripheral tissues or by both?

4.1.3. Experimental studies: In animals, McCaleb et al (42) demonstrated that 20 hour exposure of rat adipocytes to sulphonylureas markedly increased their sensitivity to insulin but with no change in insulin receptor activity, suggesting a direct intracellular locus for the extrapancreatic effects. Amatruda et al (43) also showed a direct effect of tolazamide on enchancing insulin induced lipogenesis in cultured hepatocytes from normal and diabetic rats. However, in vivo insulin treatment per se also restores hepatocyte insulin sensitivity so that there may be both a direct and indirect sulphonylurea effect on tissue insulin responsiveness. Using isotopic methods for estimating the relative contributions of hepatic glucose output and tissue glucose consumption to the basal fasting level of glycaemia in human non-insulin-dependent diabetics, Defronzo and Simonson (44) demonstrated a 27% reduction in hepatic glucose output after 3 months' treatment with glyburide, the hepatic glucose output correlating strongly with fasting blood glucose concentration. Although sulphonylurea administration did not change the basal glucose disposal rate, it enhanced insulin-mediated glucose metabolism and, in diabetics, increased B-cell responsiveness (45). Kolterman and Olefsky (46) have also demonstrated both reduction of hepatic glucose output and increase in insulin-mediated peripheral glucose metabolism after 3 and 28 months of sulphonylurea treatment in man with evidence of effects at both receptor and postreceptor loci. This conclusion was essentially endorsed by Mandarino and Gerich (47) though they view the principal long-term effect of sulphonylureas as being attributable to reduction of post-receptor resistance to insulin action in peripheral rather than hepatic tissue. They also stress the 'heterogeneity' of the mechanisms responsible for the chronic glucose intolerance of NIDDM. Their finding of comparatively trivial effects of sulphonylurea administration on receptor specific insulin binding contrasts with the substantial increase in monocyte insulin binding provoked in vivo in both NIDDM patients and normal controls and directly in vitro by sulphonylureas by Beck-Nielsen et al (48) to which they are inclined to attribute the major part of extrapancreatic sulphonylurea effect.
Serial euglycaemic clamp studies (49) of 7 IDDM patients showed no change in insulin requirement to maintain a plasma glucose of 6.7 mmol/L either during a concomitant tolbutamide infusion or after 6 days of 2.5 g/day of tolbutamide by mouth. While this study does not exclude the unlikely possibility of opposing changes in hepatic versus peripheral sensitivity to insulin, it suggests that sulphonylureas are unlikely to be a useful adjunct to insulin in the treatment of IDDM. These findings support the clinical studies of Grunberger et al (50) and of Ward et al (51) despite the evidence in vitro of sulphonylurea enhancement of insulin effects on isolated tissues - adipocytes, skeletal muscle and liver cell membrane insulin

receptors. Burke et al (52) showed that the addition of glibenclamide significantly improved mean daily glycaemia in IDDM patients who retained some insulin secretory capacity on the basis of fasting plasma C-peptide values > 0.07 mmol/L. These patients were rather better controlled in any case and it seems doubtful whether the statistically significant but quantitatively small glycaemic improvement was clinically significant. Since some non-secretors also showed a fall in insulin requirement, they suggest there may also be a non-pancreatic effect in addition to B-cell stimulation. Pfeiffer et al (53) however have reported that the pancreatic action of sulphonylureas persists after chronic treatment and that it still accounts for the main hypoglycaemic action of these drugs during long term treatment.

4.2. Other effects and side effects of sulphonylureas

In addition to their common hypoglycaemic action, the sulphonylureas have other effects and side-effects, some of which are peculiar to individual drugs rather than the group as a whole. Acetohexamide, tolazamide and to a lesser degree glyburide have a mild diuretic effect (54). By contrast, chlorpropamide (55) has an antidiuretic action due to potentiation or possibly increased secretion of antidiuretic hormone (ADH). The effect is rarely clinically important and tends to affect elderly patients receiving large doses of chlorpropamide for prolonged periods (56). The antidiuretic effect of chlorpropamide has been applied therapeutically in controlling lesser degrees of diabetes insipidus.

Chlorpropamide also has the special property in many subjects of causing alcohol-induced flushing, rarely if ever seen with other sulphonylureas. The chlorpropamide alcohol flush' (CPAF) phenomenon, first recognised soon after chlorpropamide was introduced (57, 58), aroused considerable interest following the suggestion that it could be a genetic marker for a major subgroup of NIDDM (59) and also that it was a prognostic indicator of relative freedom from diabetic complications (60-62). Leslie & Pyke (59) devised a 'single challenge test' of 250mg of chlorpropamide followed 30 mins later by 40mls of sherry. They reported a positive CPAF response in 51% of NIDDM patients (in 81% when there was a family history of NIDDM), compared to only 10% of IDDM patients and 10% of non-diabetic volunteers. However other investigators have found CPAF rates in NIDDM varying between 4% and 40% (63-65). In a double-blind, randomised placebo-controlled epidemiological study, we (66) could find no significant difference in CPAF rates in non-diabetics (6.2%), IDDM patients (9.7%) or NIDDM patients (10.5%), whether there was a family history of diabetes or not. However, our study showed a much higher CPAF rate (56%) in NIDDM patients who were chronically receiving chlorpropamide therapeutically, and who therefore had high 'background' plasma chlorpropamide levels.

The importance of a high plasma chlorpropamide level was demonstrated by showing that 70% of IDDM patients and 80% of NIDDM patients who were CPAF negative when tested after a single dose of chlorpropamide became positive after raising plasma chlorpropamide levels with one week's pretreatment with the drug (67). These and similar findings from others (65,68) strongly suggest that plasma chlorpropamide concentration is the major determinant for CPAF. The high CPAF rate originally reported by Leslie & Pyke (59) was probably a consequence of the fact that the majority of their NIDDM patients were chronically treated with chlorpropamide (69). A high CPAF rate in IDDM patients and even in normal subjects following multiple doses of chlorpropamide has recently been reported by Pyke's group (70,71). Our studies (Table III & IV) and those of other investigators (72-74) have also failed to show any association between a positive single dose or multiple dose CPAF test and a reduced risk of small or large vessel disease.

Other side effects of sulphonylureas are uncommon and include allergic skin rashes and gastrointestinal sysmptoms. Hypoglycaemia has been recorded with all sulphonylureas but the risk is higher with the more potent preparations such as glibenclamide (75) or with chlorpropamide which has a long biological half-life. Overdosage, displacement from protein binding by other drugs, use in patients with renal or liver disease, failure to supervise response and adjust dosage as weight falls, long fasts, especially after rigorous exertion and the use of long acting preparations in elderly patients increase the risk of sulphonylurea-induced hypoglycaemia.

TABLE III: FREQUENCY OF VASCULAR COMPLICATIONS IN CPAF *

	CPAF +ve (n=40)	CPAF -ve (n=344)
RETINOPATHY		
Background only	24.0 %	20.6 %
Maculopathy	12.0 %	5.9 %
Proliferative	8.0 %	3.9 %
PROTEINURIA	12.5 %	15.1 %
MACROVASCULAR DISEASE		
Angina	15.0 %	15.7 %
Myocardial infarct	7.5 %	8.4 %
Intermittent claudication	5.0 %	6.7 %
Hypertension	27.5 %	30.5 %
Stroke	5.0	5.2
Any type	37.5	41.9

* Single dose CPAF test. Difference between the two groups not significant (p > 0.05) for each observation

TABLE IV: FREQUENCY OF RETINOPATHY IN CPAF +ve
AND -ve DIABETICS AFTER 7 DAYS OF CHLORPROPAMIDE

	CPAF +ve (n=45)	CPAF -ve (n=14)
RETINOPATHY ABSENT	64.4 %	57.1 %
RETINOPATHY PRESENT	35.5 %	42.9 %
. Background only	20.0 %	35.7 %
. Maculopathy	8.9 %	7.2 %
. Proliferative	6.7 %	0.0 %

Difference between the two groups not significant
($p > 0.05$) for each observation.

5.1 BIGUANIDES

The biguanides differ from the sulphonylureas both in chemical structure (Table II) and mode of action. Metformin is the only one commonly used nowadays. Unlike the sulphonylureas, the biguanides do not' stimulate insulin secretion from pancreatic islets; their hypoglycaemic action seen only in patients with NIDDM (76) is probably entirely extrapancreatic. Various mechanisms of action have been proposed, including (a) reduction of glucose absorption from the gastrointestinal tract (77), (b) depression of appetite (78), (c) inhibition of gluconeogenesis in the liver with resultant decrease in hepatic glucose output (79) and (d) stimulation of glucose uptake in peripheral tissues (80). An increase in binding of insulin to its tissue receptors by metformin has also been observed in vitro and in vivo studies by some investigators (81) but not confirmed by others (82).

The predominantly extrapancreatic effects of biguanides without an associated increase in insulin secretion confer certain advantages in the treatment of NIDDM, particularly in the obese patient. A modest fall in blood glucose concentration can be achieved, accompanied with a degree of weight reduction without an increase in plasma insulin levels; there is little risk of hypoglycaemia. It has also been suggested that the extrapancreatic hypoglycaemic effect of biguanides could potentiate the action of insulin in IDDM patients (83-85) and so reduce insulin requirement and hyperinsulinism, but the clinical usefulness of this remains to be assessed.

Unfortunately, the inhibitory effect of biguanides on hepatic gluconeogenesis tends to result in an increase in blood lactate concentration, with the potential though uncommon risk of life-threatening lactic acidosis (18). This complication is more likely to occur with phenformin which is concentrated and metabolised in the liver than with metformin which is not. The presence of liver disease or any condition which reduces hepatic blood flow or hepatic function increases the risk of lactic acidosis during biguanide treatment. Furthermore since these drugs are excreted by the kidneys, renal impairment increases the blood concentration of both the drug and lactate. It appears to be rarely that phenformin, used in correct dosage per se, is responsible for lactic acidosis, but that other provocative factors including renal or liver disease, alcoholism, poor tissue perfusion such as occurs after myocardial infarct or any cause of shock, are also likely to contribute to an important degree. In view of this serious, though uncommon complication, biguanides have reduced in popularity, and several countries, including Britain and the U.S.A have prohibited the use of phenformin. Metformin, which has a much lower risk of lactic acidosis (86) is still widely used (but not in USA), but the drug cannot be recommended in NIDDM patients with cardiac, renal or liver disease. Other side effects of biguanides are mainly gastrointestinal and include diarrhea, dyspepsia and nausea. They can also impair absorption of other dietary nutrients besides glucose, especially vitamin B12, though only rarely is clinical vitamin B12 deficiency observed (87).

Metformin may be considered in the management of the obese NIDDM patient whose glycaemic control is inadequate with diet alone. It has perhaps enjoyed its most useful role as an adjunct to sulphonylurea therapy if the latter does not produce adequate glycaemic control (primary failure) or if the response deteriorates after an interval (secondary failure). If hyperglycaemia is not adequately controlled with triple therapy (diet, sulphonylurea and metformin), a change to insulin therapy should not be delayed. This is usually seen in NIDDM patients who are not overweight, who present between the age of 30 and 50 years, often with metabolic symptoms and moderately elevated blood glucose levels but without ketosis.

6. OTHER HYPOGLYCAEMIC AGENTS

Salicylates and aspirin in particular have been known to possess hypoglycaemic activity and even been used as oral antidiabetic agents for over 100 years (1). The accumulation of clinical and experimental information has recently been well reviewed by Baron (88). While there seems little doubt that either alone or with other insulin secretagogues, salicylates have some blood glucose lowering activity, the mechanism remains uncertain. There appears to be a direct effect on insulin secretion in man and an adjuvant effect in sulphonylurea induced hypoglycaemia though this has been ascribed to competitive displacement of sulphonylureas from plasma protein binding (89). Peripheral effects of aspirin on glucose uptake have also been suggested. The inhibitory effects of aspirin on prostaglandin synthesis have been investigated as a possible mechanism of the metabolic effect of this versatile substance; in vitro studies suggest that this may explain enhanced early pancreatic B-cell insulin release. To achieve significant therapeutic effects plasma levels need to be high and this raises problems of gastric bleeding and systemic salicylism.

Ciglitazone,5-(4-(1-methylcyclohexylmethoxy)benzyl)-thiazolidine-2,4-dione lowers blood glucose in genetically diabetic animal models (ob/ob and db/db mice) and this is associated with increased glucose metabolism and insulin binding, reduced gluconeogenesis and regranulation of pancreatic beta cells (90). However, it is not known whether this regranulation is a direct B-cell effect or whether, by lowering blood glucose by a peripheral action, the reduced hyperglycaemic stimulus to the islet allows more normal insulin synthesis and storage. It is interesting to note that similar B-cell regranulation effect is shown in experimental diabetic animals treated with oxytetracyline.

Other non-sulphonylurea, non-biguanide hypoglycaemic agents and their postulated mode of action are summarised in Table V.

TABLE V: OTHER HYPOGLYCAEMIC AGENTS

CLASS	COMPOUND	POSTULATED ACTION	REF
Substituted pyridine	2,4-diamino-5-cyano--6-halopyridine	Insulin secretagogue	91
Substituted guanidine	McN-3495, pirogliride	?Periheral glucose uptake	92
Fatty acid analogue	McN-3716, methyl 2-tetradecylglycidate	Fatty acid oxid. inhibition(CAT)	93
Substit. alcanoic acid	B807-27	Fatty acid oxid. inhibition	94
Thiazolidinedione	Ciglitazone	Reduce insulin resistance	90
B-adrenergic agonist	TA-078	Sensitize B-cell response	95
ω-phenylvaleric acid		Inhibit gluco-neogenesis	96
Somatostatin anlogue	D-Trp^8, D-cys^{14}--somatostatin	Inhibit G.H glucagon	97
Enzyme inducer	Phenobarbitone Medroxyprogesterone	Postreceptor activation	98

7. CONCLUSIONS

As yet, oral agents are restricted to non- insulin dependent diabetics. Sulphonylureas remain the most widely used agents though not all NIDDM patients respond to them and, with time, the response is greatly reduced in those who do. The mechanism of this secondary failure to sulphonylureas is uncertain -whether it represents a specific loss of sensitivity (pancreatic and/or peripheral) to the drug or simply signals the worsening natural history of NIDDM is unknown. The question of long-term effectiveness in preventing complications remains unresolved though studies are in progress. There has been little substantiation of the UGDP reports suggesting cardiovascular toxicity. The hope that 'early diabetes' might be delayed in its progression has not been realised. Though the insulin secretory response is very likely to be mediated through translocation of calcium ions in the B-cell, it is not yet clear how this is activated. The nature of the 'extrapancreatic' effects remains obscure though it now seems more likely to be due to post-receptor events than to an effect on insulin receptors directly. Although there is a profusion of sulphonylurea preparations there appear to be few, if any, fundamental differences in their actions. Differences in dose-level potencies and duration of action are attributable to variations in substituent radicals attached to the sulphonylurea core. The risk of lactic acidosis with the biguanides has largely restricted their use to metformin only. The latter has comparatively limited hypoglycaemic potency and is often used to bolster the failing sulphonylurea action. A number of alternative blood glucose lowering preparations are currently being investigated. These are at a number of points in the pathways of glucose metabolism and their therapeutic potential, either alone or in combination with other drugs, remains to be defined.

Whatever oral therapy is used it remains of major importance in diabetic management to treat the patient comprehensively, paying particular attention to the prevention of vascular disease by energetic control of the common risk factors - raised blood pressure, hyperlipidaemia, cigarette smoking, obesity and physical inactivity.

ACKNOWLEDGMENT

We thank Dr N. Morrish for his assistance during the preparation of this chapter. Dr S. Ng Tang Fui was supported by Novo Laboratories, Basingstoke, England.

REFERENCES

01. Ebstein W, Muller J. 1876. Berl Klin Wochenschr 13: 53-56.
02. Frank E, Nothmann M, Wagner A. 1926. Dtsch Med Wochenschr 52: 2067-2107.
03. Loubatieres A. In Volk BW & Wellman KF (Eds). The Diabetic Pancreas. Plenum Press. N. York 1977, P489-515.
04. Franke E, Fuchs J. 1955. Dtsch Med Wochenschr 80: 1449-1452.
05. Krall LP, Camerini-Davalos R. 1957. Proc Soc Exper Biol & Med 95: 345.
06. Levine R, Duncan GC. 1956. Metabolism 5: 721-829.
07. Goldner MG (Ed). 1959. Ann NY Acad Sci 74: 407-1028.
08. Keen H, Jarrett RJ, Mc Cartney P. 1982. Diabetologia 22: 73-78.
09. Jarrett RJ, Keen H, Grabauskas V. 1979. Diabetes Care 2: 175-186.
10. Schöffling K. Personal communication.
11. Wade O, Hadden DR, Hood H. 1973. J Prev Soc Med 27: 44-48.
12. University Group Diabetes Program. 1970. Diabetes (Suppl) 19:789-830.
13. Kilo C, Miller JP, Williamson JR. 1980. JAMA 243: 430-457.
14. Pasikivi J. 1970. Acta Med Scand (Suppl) 507: 1-82.
15. Keen H, Jarrett RJ, Fuller JH. 1974. International Congress Series 312. Excerpta Medica . Amsterdam P588-601.
16. Carlstrom S, Persson G, Schersten B. 1975. Diabetes (Suppl 2) 24: 414.
17. Ohneda A, Maruhama Y, Itabashi H et al. 1978. J Exp Med 222: 205-222.
18. Editorial. 1977. Br Med J 2: 1436.
19. Levey GS, Palmer RF, Lasseter KC et al. 1971. J Clin Endocrinol Metab 33: 371-374.
20. Curtis GP, Setchfield J, Lucchesi BR. 1975. J Pharm Exp Ther 194: 264-273.
21. Young JL(Jr), Burr IM, Perry JM et al. 1975. Am Heart J 89: 189-194.
22. Turner RC for Multi-centre Study Group. 1983. Diabetologia 24: 404-411.
23. Holman RR, Turner RC. 1977. Lancet 1: 469-474.
24. Peacock I, Tattersall RB. 1984. Lancet 1: 469-474.
25. Yallow RS, Black H, Villazon M, Berson SA. 1960. Diabetes 18: 356-362.
26. Duckworth WC, Solomon SS, Kitabchi AE. 1972. J Clin Endocrinol Metab 35: 585-591.
27. Lebovitz HE, Feinglos MN, Bucholtz HK, Lebovitz FL. 1977. J Clin Endocrinol Metab 45: 601-604.
28. Greenfield M, Doberns L, Rosenthal M et al. 1982. Diabetes 31: 307-312.
29. Loubatieres A. 1946. Arch Intern Physiol 54: 174-177.
30. Mirsky IA, Perisutti G, Jinks R. 1956. Proc Soc Exp Biol Med 91: 475-477
31. Bressler R, Jackson J. 1981. Drugs 22: 211-245.
32. Duncan L, Baird J. 1960. Pharmacol Rev 12: 91-158.
33. Helman B, Selhin J, Taljedal IB. 1973. Diabetologia 9: 210-216.
34. Kloppel G, Schafer J. 1976. Diabetologia 12: 227-234.
35. Grodsky GM, Epstein GH, Franska R, Karam JH. 1977. Fed Proc 36: 2714-2719.
36. Gylfe E, Hellman J, Sehlin J, Taljedal IB. 1984. Experientia 40: 1126-1135.
37. Aschcroft FM, Harrison DE, Ashcroft SJH. 1985. Nature (In press).
38. Schauder P, Frerich H. 1975. Diabetologia 11: 301-305.
39. Judzewitsch RG, Pffeifer MA, Best JD et al. 1982. J Clin Endocrinol & Metab 55: 321-328.
40. Reaven G, Dray J. 1967. Diabetes 16: 487-492.
41. Singer DL, Hurwitz. 1967. N Engl J Med 277: 450-456.
42. Mc Caleb ML, Maloof BL, Nowak SM, Lockwood DH. 1984. Diabetes Care 7 (Suppl 1): 42-46.
43. Amatruda JM, Salhanick AI, Chang CL. 1984. Diabetes Care 7(Suppl 1): 42.

44. De Fronzo RA, Simonson DC. 1984. Diabetes Care 7 (Suppl 1): 72-80.
45. Simonson DC, Ferrannini E, Bevilacqua S et al. 1984. Diabetes Care 33: 838-845.
46. Kolterman OG, Olefsky JM. 1984. Diabetes Care 7 (Suppl 1): 81-88.
47. Mandarino LJ, Gerich JE. 1984. Diabetes Care 7 (Suppl 1): 89-99.
48. Beck-Nielsen H, Hjollund E, Pedersen O et al. 1984. Diabetes Care 7 (Suppl 1): 100-105.
49. Ratzmann KP, Schulz B, Heinke P, Besch W. 1984. Diabetologia 27: 8-12.
50. Gruneberger G, Ryan J, Gorden PH. 1982. Diabetes Care 31: 890-896.
51. Ward EA, Ward GM, Turner RC. 1981. Br Med J 283: 278.
52. Burke BJ, Hartog M, Waterfield MR, 1984. Acta Endocrinol 107: 70-77.
53. Pfeiffer MA, Halter RG, Judzewitsch RG et al. 1984. Diabetes Care 7 (Suppl 1): 25-34.
54. Moses AM, Howaritz J, Miller M. 1973. Ann Intern Med 78: 541-544.
55. Weissman PN, Shenkman L, Gregerman RI. 1971. N Engl J Med 284: 65-71.
56. Kadowaki T, Hagura R, Kajinuma H et al. 1983. Diabetes Care 6: 468-471.
57. Cardonnet LJ, Staffieri JJ, Eberhart DR et al. 1959. Ann NY Acad Sci 74: 771-787.
58. Signorelli S. 1959. Ann NY Acad Sc 74: 900-903.
59. Leslie RDG, Pyke DA. 1978. Br Med J 1: 1519-1521.
60. Leslie RDG, Barnett AH, Pyke DA. 1979. Lancet 1: 997-999.
61. Barnett AH, Leslie RDG, Pyke D. 1981. Br Med J 282: 522-523.
62. Barnett AH, Pyke DA, 1980. Br Med J 2: 261-262.
63. Kobberling J, Bengsch N, Bruggeboes B et al. 1980. Diabetologia 19: 359 -363.
64. De Silva NE, Tunbridge WMG, Alberti KGMM. 1981. Lancet 1: 128-131.
65. Jerntorp P, Almer LO, Melander A. 1981. Lancet 1: 165-166.
66. Ng Tang Fui S, Keen H, Jarrett RJ et al. 1983. Br Med J. 287: 1509-1512.
67. Ng Tang Fui S, Keen H, Jarrett RJ et al. 1983. N Engl J Med 309: 93-96.
68. Pontiroli AE, De Pasqua A, Colombo R et al. 1983. Act Diab Lat 20: 117-123.
69. Leslie RDG, Pyke DA. 1982. In Diabetes and its late complications. Cudworth A, Andreani D, Bodansky HJ, Squadrilo G (Eds). J Libbey. London P 32-37.
70. Wiles P, Pyke DA. 1984. Clinical Science 67: 375-381.
71. Volkmann HP, Hoskins PJ, Wiles P, Pyke DA. 1985(Abstract). British Diabetic Association Medical and Scientific Section Spring Meeting. Oxford. 28-30 March.
72. Ng Tang Fui S. 1985. MD Thesis. Univ of London . Submitted.
73. Radder JK, Box MC, Lemkes HM. 1980. Lancet 2: 1037.
74. Mann JI, Houston. 1983. In Diabetes and Epidemiological Perspectives. Mann JI, Pyorala K, Teuscher A (Eds). Churchill Livingstone. Edinburgh & London. P 147-153.
75. Asplund K, Wilhom BE, Lithner. 1983. Diabetologia 24: 412-417.
76. Fajans SS, Moorhouse JA, Doorenbos et al . 1960. Diabetes 9: 194-201.
77. Czyzyk A, Tawecki J, Sadowski J, Sczepanik Z. 1968. Diabetes 17:492-496.
78. Patel DP, Stowers JM. 1964. Lancet 2: 282-284.
79. Meyer F, Ipacktchi M, Clauser H. 1967. Nature 213: 203-204.
80. Butterfield WJH, Whichelow MJ. 1968. Lancet 2: 785-788.
81. Vigneri R, Gullo D, PezzinoV. 1984. Diabetes Care 7 (Suppl 1):113-117.
82. Prager R, Schernthaner . 1983. Diabetes 32: 1083-1086.
83. Pagano G, Tagliafero V, Carta Q et al. 1983. Diabetologia 24: 351-354.
84. Gin H, Slama G, Weissbrodt et al. 1982. Diabetologia. 23: 34-36.
85. Coscelli MD, Palmari V, Saccardi et al. 1984. Curr Ther Res 35: 1058-1069.

86. Luft D, Schmulling RM, Eggstein M. 1978. Diabetologia. 14: 75-78.
87. Adams JF, Clark JS, Ireland JT et al. 1983. Diabetologia 24: 16-18.
88. Baron SH. 1982. Diabetes Care. 5: 64-71.
89. Stowers JM, Constable LW, Hunter RB. 1959. Ann NY ACad Sci. 74: 689-695
90. Chang AY, Wyse BM, Gilchrist BJ et al. 1983. Diabetes 32: 830-839.
91. Johnson DG , de Haen C. 1979. Mol Pharmacol 15: 287-293.
92. Tutwiler GF, Kirsch T, Bridi G. 1978. Diabetes 27: 856-876.
93. Tutwiler GF, Dellevigne P. 1979. J Biol Chem 254: 2935-2941.
94. Wolf HPO, Eistetter K, Ludwig G. 1982. Diabetologia 22: 456-463.
95. Awai H, Inamasu M, Totsuka T et al. 1983. Biochem Pharmac 32: 849-855.
96. De Galdeano LG, Bressler R, Brendel K. 1973. J Biol Chem 28: 2514-2520.
97. Meyers C, Arimura A, Gordin A et al. 1977. Biochem Biophy Res Commun 74: 630-636.
98. Sotaniemi EA, Arranto AJ, Sutinen S et al. 1983. Clin Pharmacol Ther 33: 826-835.

2.2. Insulin

2.2.1. Introduction: Insulin treatment

J. Terpstra

When, in 1922, insulin was discovered, all thoughts circled around its life-saving quality. After a few decades, however, it became clear that severe long-term complications of diabetes developed in insulin treated patients and that, although mortality from diabetic coma decreased, mortality and morbidity from micro- and macrovascular disease increased. Many studies were carried out in order to investigate whether good control of diabetes might prevent the development of these distressing complications. Unfortunately useful parameters to estimate good or bad control were lacking.

Today the advocacy of normoglycaemia is better founded than formerly could be possible. In the first place accurate estimates of blood glucose values became within the scope of patients, who thus were enabled to control their own blood glucose levels. In a number of patients insulin infusion pumps became the expedients to keep blood glucose levels within normal ranges. Finally HbA1c values allow a reasonably accurate estimate of mean blood glucose levels over a longer period of time. However, it now becomes apparent that, in maintaining normal peripheral blood glucose levels, these patients develop peripheral hyperinsulinaemia.

In non-diabetics, peripheral hyperinsulinaemia is encountered in obese people. Here the stimulating effect of insulin on the glucose uptake in adipose tissue is diminished. This is compensated by an increased insulin production, so that normoglycaemia can be maintained.

Non-insulin dependent diabetics are generally obese and thus insulin resistant. Evidence piles up that in these diabetics the secretion of insulin by the B-cell is also defective, especially in its response to glucose. Later on these patients often become insulin deficient.

Regarding the state of hyperinsulinaemia, which can be encountered in insulin dependent as well as in non-insulin dependent diabetics, the following questions arise:
- Why does peripheral hyperinsulinaemia develop in insulin dependent normoglycaemic diabetics?
- Have these patients - or do the acquire - insulin resistance?
- Is the often encountered peripheral hyperinsulinaemia in non-insulin dependent diabetics the result of concomittant obesity? Can a delayed secretion of insulin, as probably occurs in these patients, cause peripheral hyperinsulinaemia?
- Has peripheral hyperinsulinaemia clinical consequences?

Although peripheral plasma insulin levels may be higher than normal in well controlled insulin dependent normoglycaemic diabetics, portal levels are lower. Hepatic glucose production is inhibited by insulin.

Low insulin levels in the portal system, therefore, have a relatively decreased inhibiting effect on hepatic glucose production, thereby causing a relative increase in peripheral blood glucose levels. The normalization of these levels may require a higher than normal peripheral insulin level. This brings us to the possible effects of high peripheral insulin levels together with a greater than normal glucose supply to peripheral tissues. The latter may also have consequences for cellular function and survival, as some of these tissues (for instance endothelium) have an active sorbitol pathway.

In diabetics, insulin is commonly injected peripherally, which means that in first instance the liver is by-passed. In most cases of pancreas transplantation the transplant does not drain on the portal vein. The site of the insulin supply therefore should be carefully considered, the more so because pancreas transplantation in diabetics seems to become a real therapeutic possibility.

The following questions arise:
- Would portal insulin delivery in insulin dependent diabetics prevent the development of peripheral hyperinsulinaemia?
- Is it advisable to aim at portal (or peritoneal) delivery of insulin?

Insulin infusion pumps have made it possible to deliver insulin continuously, day and night, imitating the basal insulin secretion in healthy people. There are indications that in normals basal insulin secretion is a pulsatile process, the interval between the pulses being approximately 10 to 15 minutes. In pump-treated patients it depends on the quality of the pump how often, and in which quantities, insulin can be delivered. Insulin in these patients, moreover, is commonly injected subcutaneously, and not intraportally.

- Does it make sense to deliver insulin in a pulsatile way when using the subcutaneous route? If so, is the time interval between the pulses important?
- What are the effects of pulsatile intraportal insulin delivery as compared with continuous delivery? Should we aim at intraportal pulsatile insulin delivery?

In the following chapters, part of the above raised questions will be considered and discussed.

2.2.2. Hyperinsulinaemia
E.R. Trimble

Hyperinsulinaemia arises spontaneously under many different circumstances and can be induced experimentally by a variety of means. The consequences of hyperinsulinaemia are complex and depend to some extent on its aetiology.

Hyperinsulinaemia may arise from primary overproduction of insulin as occurs in nesidioblastosis and in insulinomas (1). The latter may be sporadic or occur as part of the autosomal dominant multiple endocrine adenoma syndrome type I (2). Overproduction of insulin also occurs in many conditions associated with insulin resistance. Such resistance may rarely occur as a manifestation of a primary insulin receptor defect (3), or in equally rare cases where there are antibodies to the insulin receptor (4,5). Endogenous hyperinsulinaemia occurs most frequently in association with the insulin resistance of obesity (6); some subjects may also have type II diabetes. Insulin resistance also occurs in association with glucocorticoid excess (7), acromegaly (8), leprechaunism (9), myotonic dystrophy (10), spinal cord injury (11), and lesions of the ventromedial hypothalamus (12). Insulin is eliminated by the liver and kidney (13,14), and major insufficiency of these organs normally leads to hyperinsulinaemia due in part to reduced catablism but also to a certain degree of associated insulin resistance (15,16). Apparent hyperinsulinaemia may occur as a radioimmunoassay artefact in familial hyperproinsulinaemia. In this condition an abnormal amino acid occurs at the site of cleavage of C-peptide thus rendering this site resistant to the usual cleaving enzymes. Since proinsulin has a markedly reduced metabolic effectiveness with respect to insulin the pancreatic β-cell is stimulated to produce more and "hyperinsulinaemia" occurs, often associated with diabetes mellitus (17,18). Similarly, stimulation of overproduction seems to occur with mutant insulins of low metabolic effectiveness (19,20). In both of these syndromes the affected subjects will respond normally to exogenous insulin. Finally, hyperinsulinaemia may be due to exogenous insulin and is the usual finding in insulin-treated diabetic subjects. More rarely it is found in cases of the Munchausen syndrome (21). In both of these conditions there will be an abnormally low C-peptide: insulin ratio in peripheral blood

with C-peptide being absent in type I diabetic subjects.
(Since C-peptide is mainly eliminated by the kidney, a high
C-peptide:insulin ratio may occur in renal failure).

Many cell types are insulin sensitive such as the hepatocyte, myocyte, adipocyte, fibroblast, and the pancreatic
acinar cell, etc. The overall effect of hyperinsulinaemia will
depend on factors such as the degree of hyperinsulinaemia, the
time during which hyperinsulinaemia persists and the background against which it arises. The actions of insulin are
multiple and often require different insulin concentrations.
For example, while the antilipolytic effect of insulin may be
seen in vitro at an insulin concentration of $10^{-11}M$, stimulation of amino acid transport in hepatocytes will require a
slightly higher concentration and stimulation of DNA synthesis
may be best seen at 10^{-8} or $10^{-7}M$. From the point of view of
time, there are also marked differences with stimulation of
glucose uptake occurring within seconds, whereas the effects
of insulin on DNA synthesis can only be seen after some hours.
If hyperinsulinaemia arises on the background of hepatic or
renal failure then the signs of hyperinsulinaemia may be
totally swamped by the signs of the primary illness. Similarly, the background presence or absence of insulin resistance
will determine the effectiveness of insulin in producing any
of its well described actions, e.g. its effects on amino acid
metabolism and glucose disposal (22).

Clinically the most frequent cases of hyperinsulinaemia are
seen in obesity (with or without type II diabetes) and in
treated type I diabetes, with insulinoma being much more rare.
These conditions are frequently associated with insulin resistance and downregulation of insulin receptors. One of the most
debated subjects in this area is the question of the (causal?)
relationship between hyperinsulinaemia, insulin receptor number and insulin resistance. In many instances, especially in
obesity, there is an inverse relationship between the plasma
insulin concentration and the insulin receptor number. The
literature is voluminous on this subject, but there are now
too many notable exceptions for this to be taken as a general-
ization (see ref. 23 for minireview). Similarly, although at
one time downregulation of insulin receptors was taken as
being synonymous with insulin resistance, this is now known
not to be the case. Furthermore, insulin resistance develops
at different rates in different tissues and in various metabolic pathways within the same tissue. Some illustrations will
be given centred on the liver or hepatocyte. In type I
diabetes, while peripheral tissues have been found to be insulin resistant in most (24-27) but not all (28) series investigated, it would appear that the liver remains very sensitive
to the inhibitory action of insulin on glucose production
(29-30). (It should be remembered that in insulin-treated
type I diabetes the plasma insulin levels are rarely

unphysiologically high for the liver). On the other hand, in the well established hyperinsulinaemia of the obese Zucker rat resistance to insulin has been demonstrated not only in the peripheral tissues but also in the liver (31). In the case of insulinomas, although downregulation of insulin receptors (32) and peripheral insulin resistance (33) occur, the clinically most important factor in determining glucose homeostasis in vivo remains the inhibition by insulin of glucose production by the liver (33). When isolated hepatocytes are exposed to near physiological concentrations of insulin in vitro downregulation of insulin receptors occurs (34,35). However, within the hepatocyte there are divergent effects of such exposure to insulin on different metabolic pathways. Thus, there is no change in sensitivity and even an increase in maximum responsiveness of insulin-induced lipogenesis, while a reduced sensitivity of insulin-stimulated amino acid uptake [also the case for cultured human fibroblasts (36)] follows the exposure to insulin (35). From the above it is clear that exposure to physiological or supraphysiological concentrations of insulin does not affect each insulin sensitive pathway to the same extent and that under certain conditions downregulation of insulin receptors can even be associated with increased responsiveness in some pathways (35). Hyperinsulinaemia is often found in cirrhosis. Under such circumstances there may be no change in insulin binding either to circulating monocytes (37) or to isolated adipocytes (38) and although insulin sensitivity is reduced, maximal insulin responsiveness is actually increased both in vivo (37) and in vitro in the isolated adipocyte (38). In completely different situations downregulation of insulin receptors may be associated with decreased responsiveness in tissues (39) and decreased responsiveness may occur without alteration of receptors (40). Downregulation of insulin receptors involves a decrease in the number of receptors in the plasma membrane without a decrease in the total receptor number per cell. In the downregulated state more receptors are found in the intracellular pool than under basal conditions (41). Another variable is the rate at which insulin resistance may occur within different metabolic pathways of the same tissue, e.g. muscle (42). There is a further interesting dimension to the modulation of insulin receptor number. It has been found that hydrogen peroxide, wheat germ agglutinin, vitamin K_5, and other substances can mimic some of the effects of insulin on target tissues (43). These substances do not acutely interfere with insulin binding. However, when tissue is preincubated with such insulin mimickers, downregulation of the insulin receptor occurs. This means that insulin binding can be modulated by post-receptor events without the necessity for changes in ambient insulin concentrations. It has become clear from several recent studies that even in those conditions where insulin resistance eventually arises in the presence of hyperinsulinaemia there may be an early period of normal or even enhanced responsiveness to insulin. These studies have been carried out following induction of hyperinsulinaemia in man or laboratory animals, or by the study of very early time points in genetically determined obesity syndromes in animals (12, 44-47).

Although there remains much uncertainty about the pathophysiological relationships among hyperinsulinaemia, insulin receptor number and insulin resistance there is no doubt that hyperinsulinaemia is undesirable. Several recent prospective studies have shown a positive correlation between hyperinsulinaemia and atherosclerosis, a relationship which was independent of other risk factors (see 48 for review). Similarly, it has been shown that hyperinsulinaemia, even in the absence of increased levels of substrates, can lead to the development of foetal macrosomia and increased birth weight (49). For these and other reasons it is clearly desirable to reduce hyperinsulinaemia by food restriction or exercise in the obese and by better timing of insulin administration in the diabetic (50).

REFERENCES

1. Fajans SS & Floyd JC Jr.: Diagnosis and management of insulinomas. Ann. Rev. Med. 30:313, 1979.
2. Schimke RN: Syndromes with multiple endocrine gland involvement. Prog. Med. Genet. 3:143, 1979.
3. Scarlett JA, Kolterman OG, Moore P, Saekow M, Insel J, Griffin J, Mako M, Rubenstein AH & Olefsky JM: Insulin resistance and diabetes due to a genetic defect in insulin receptors. J. Clin. Endocrinol. Metab. 55:123, 1982.
4. Flier JS, Kahn CR, Roth J & Bar RS: Antibodies that impair insulin receptor binding in an unusual diabetic syndrome with severe insulin resistance. Science 190:63, 1975.
5. Kahn CR, Flier JS, Bar RS, Archer JA, Gorden P, Martin MM, & Roth J: The syndromes of insulin resistance and acanthosis nigricans-insulin-receptor disorders in man. N. Engl. J. Med. 294:739, 1976.
6. Olefsky J, Reaven GM & Farquhar JW: Effects of weight reduction on obesity. J. Clin. Invest. 53:64, 1974.
7. Caro JF & Amatruda JM: Glucocorticoid-induced insulin resistance. J. Clin. Invest. 69:866, 1982.
8. Trimble ER, Atkinson AB, Buchanan KD & Hadden DR: Plasma glucagon and insulin concentrations in acromegaly. J. Clin. Endocrinol. Metab. 51:626, 1980.
9. Kobayashi M, Olefsky JM, Elders J, Mako ME, Given BD, Schedwie HK, Fiser RH, Hintz RL, Horner JA & Rubenstein A: Insulin resistance due to a defect distal to the insulin receptor: demonstration in a patient with leprechaunism. Proc. Natl. Acad. Sci. (USA) 75:3469, 1978.
10. Kobayashi M, Meek JC & Streib E: The insulin receptor in myotonic dystrophy. J. Clin. Endocrinol. Metab. 45:821, 1977.
11. Duckworth WC, Solomon SS, Jallepalli P, Heckemeyer C, Finnern J & Powers A: Glucose intolerance due to insulin resistance in patients with spinal cord injuries. Diabetes 29:906, 1980.
12. Le Marchand-Brustel Y, Freychet P & Jeanrenaud B: Longitudinal study on the establishment of insulin resistance in hypothalamic obese mice. Endocrinology 102:74, 1978.
13. Ferrannini E, Wahren J, Faber OK, Felig P, Binder C & DeFronzo RA: Splanchnic and renal metabolism of insulin in human subjects: a dose-response study. Am. J. Physiol. 244:E517, 1983.
14. Rabkin R, Ryan MP & Duckworth WC: The renal metabolism of insulin. Diabetologia 27:351, 1984.
15. Maloff BL, McCaleb ML & Lockwood DH: Cellular basis of insulin resistance in chronic uremia. Am. J. Physiol. 245: E178, 1983.

16. Kauffman JM & Caro JF: Insulin resistance in uremia. Characterization of insulin action, binding and processing in isolated hepatocytes from chronic uremic rats. J. Clin. Invest. 71:698, 1983.
17. Gabbay KH, De Luca K, Fischer JN Jr., Mako ME & Rubenstein AH: Familial proinsulinemia: an autosomal dominant defect. N. Engl. J. Med. 294:911, 1976.
18. Robbins DC, Blix PM, Rubenstein AH, Kanazawa Y, Kosaka K & Tager HS: A human proinsulin variant at arginine 65. Nature 291:679, 1981.
19. Tager H, Given B, Baldwin D, Mako M, Markese J, Rubenstein A, Olefsky J, Kobayashi M, Kolterman O & Poucher R: A structurally abnormal insulin causing human diabetes. Nature 281:122, 1979.
20. Olefsky JM, Saekow M, Tager H & Rubenstein AH: Characterization of a mutant human insulin species. J. Biol. Chem. 255:6098, 1980.
21. Couropmitree C, Freinkel N, Nagel TC, Horwitz DL, Metzger BE, Rubenstein AH & Hahnel R: Plasma C-peptide and diagnosis of factitious hyperinsulinism. Ann. Intern. Med. 82:201, 1975.
22. Felig P, Marliss EB & Cahill GF Jr.: Plasma amino acid levels and insulin secretion in obesity. N. Engl. J. Med. 281:811, 1969.
23. Amatruda JM, Newmeyer HW & Chang CL: Insulin-induced alterations in insulin binding and insulin action in primary cultures of rat hepatocytes. Diabetes 31:145, 1982.
24. Harano Y, Ohgaku S, Kosugi K, Yasuda H, Nakano T, Kobayashi M, Hidaka H, Izumi K, Kashiwagi A, Shigeta Y: Clinical significance of altered insulin sensitivity in diabetes mellitus assessed by glucose, insulin and somatostatin infusion. J. Clin. Endocrinol. Metab. 52:982, 1981.
25. De Fronzo RA, Hendler R & Simonson D: Insulin resistance is a prominent feature of insulin-dependent diabetes. Diabetes 31:795, 1982.
26. Pernet A, Trimble ER, Kuntschen F, Damoiseaux P, Assal J.-Ph., Hahn C & Renold AE: Insulin resistance in type I (insulin-dependent) diabetes: dependence on plasma insulin concentration. Diabetologia 26:255, 1984.
27. Yki-Järvinen H & Koivisto VA: Continuous subcutaneous insulin infusion therapy decreases insulin resistance in type I diabetes. J. Clin. Endocrinol. Metab. 58:659, 1984.
28. Revers RR, Kolterman OG, Scarlett JA, Gray RS & Olefsky JM: Lack of in vivo insulin resistance in controlled insulin-dependent, type I, diabetic patients. J. Clin. Endocrinol. Metab. 58:353, 1984.
29. Sacca L, Sherwin R, Hendler R & Felig P: Influence of continuous physiologic hyperinsulinemia on glucose kinetics and counterregulatory hormones in normal and diabetic humans. J. Clin. Invest. 63:849, 1979.

30. Proietto J, Nankervis A, Aitken P, Caruso G & Alford F: Glucose utilization in type I (insulin-dependent) diabetes: evidence for a defect not reversible by acute elevations of insulin. Diabetologia 25:331, 1983.
31. Terrettaz J & Jeanrenaud B: In vivo hepatic and peripheral insulin resistance in genetically obese (fa/fa) rats. Endocrinology 112:1346, 1983.
32. Bar RS, Gorden P, Roth J & Siebert CW: Insulin receptors in patients with insulinomas: changes in receptor affinity and concentration. J. Clin. Endocrinol. Metab. 44:1210, 1977.
33. Rizza RA, Haymond MW, Verdonk CA, Mandarino LJ, Miles JM, Service FJ & Gerich JE: Pathogenesis of hypoglycemia in insulinoma patients. Diabetes 30:377, 1981.
34. Blackard WG, Guzelian PS & Small ME: Downregulation of insulin receptors in primary cultures of adult rat hepatocytes in monolayer. Endocrinology 103:548, 1978.
35. Amatruda JM, Newmeyer HW & Chang CL: Insulin-induced alterations in insulin binding and insulin action in primary cultures of rat hepatocytes. Diabetes 31:145, 1982.
36. Martin MS & Pohl SL: Insulin-induced insulin resistance of α -aminoisobutyric acid transport in cultured human skin fibroblasts. J. Biol. Chem. 254:9976, 1979.
37. Proietto J, Nankervis A, Aitken P, Dudley FJ, Caruso G & Alford FP: Insulin resistance in cirrhosis: evidence for a post-receptor defect. Clin. Endocrinol. 21:677, 1984.
38. Harewood MS, Proietto J, Dudley F & Alford FP: Insulin action and cirrhosis: insulin binding and lipogenesis in isolated adipocytes. Metabolism 31:1241, 1982.
39. Kolterman OG, Insel J, Saekow M & Olefsky JM: Mechanisms of insulin resistance in human obesity. J. Clin. Invest. 65:1272, 1980.
40. Mandarino L, Baker B, Rizza R, Genest J & Gerich J: Infusion of insulin impairs human adipocyte glucose metabolism in vitro without decreasing adipocyte insulin receptor binding. Diabetologia 27:358, 1984.
41. Krupp M & Lane MD: On the mechanism of ligand-induced downregulation of insulin receptor level in the liver cell. J. Biol. Chem. 256:1689, 1981.
42. Crettaz M, Prentki M, Zaninetti D & Jeanrenaud B: Insulin-resistance in soleus muscle from obese Zucker rats. Biochem. J. 186:525, 1980.
43. Caro JF & Amatruda JM: Insulin receptors in hepatocytes: postreceptor events mediate downregulation. Science 210:1029, 1980.
44. Doberne L, Greenfield MS, Schulz B & Reaven GM: Enhanced glucose utilization during prolonged glucose clamp studies. Diabetes 30:829, 1981.

45. Horton ES, Wardzala L, Hirshman M, Pofcher E & Horton ED: Chronic hyperinsulinemia increases insulin binding and insulin-stimulated glucose transport and metabolism in rat adipose cells without altering insulin sensitivity. Diabetes 32:25A, 1983 (abstract).

46. Trimble ER, Weir GC, Gjinovci A, Assimacopoulos-Jeannet F, Benzi R & Renold AE: Increased insulin responsiveness in vivo and in vitro consequent to induced hyperinsulinemia in the rat. Diabetes 33:444, 1984.

47. Guerre-Millo M, Lavau M, Horne JS & Wardzala LJ: Proposed mechanism for increased insulin-mediated glucose transport in adipose cells from young, obese Zucker rats. J. Biol. Chem. 260:2197, 1985.

48. Stout RW: The role of insulin in atherosclerosis in diabetics and nondiabetics. Diabetes 30 (Suppl. 2): 54, 1981.

49. Susa JB, Neave C, Sehgal P, Singer DB, Zeller WP & Schwartz R: Chronic hyperinsulinemia in the fetal rhesus monkey. Diabetes 33:656, 1984.

50. Albisser AM, Leibel BS, Ewart TG, Davidovac Z, Botz CK & Zingg W: An artificial endocrine pancreas. Diabetes 23: 389, 1974.

2.2.3. Insulin: The physiological basis of its administration
D.R. Matthews

1. BACKGROUND

Diabetes is a disease of absolute or relative insulin deficiency which may be accompanied by a variety of pathological tissue complications. These tissue complications are much rarer in non-diabetic subjects and it is therefore reasonable to assume that they are secondary to "failure" of the normal physiological homeostatic mechanisms. Such a failure is not, however, straightforward, and the markers of what we mean by "failure" are unclear. For instance, although studies have shown that complications are more likely in those with hyperglycaemia (1,2) and with longer duration (3), such findings are statistical and not absolute. Some patients may survive many years with poor control and have no complications at all. There may also be genetic susceptibility to complications as well as to developing diabetes (4), and our tendency to concentrate on hyperglycaemia as an index of poor control may be misguided. Many other body metabolites may be affected (5) and insulin itself may have adverse effects when given in inappropriate quantities, even when approximate normoglycaemia is achieved (6).

It may be that in order to prevent complications all aspects of normal physiology need to be mimicked. This may not simply mean normo-glycaemia: we may need to achieve normal intermediate metabolites (5), in the presence of normal plasma insulin concentration (7), in a ratio whch is higher in the portal system than the periphery (8), in a correct time-relationship to meals, in a fashion which can be antagonised by hypoglycaemia or stress, in a secretory pattern that can be triggered by small changes in plasma glucose. This paper examines what we might aim for and what we can achieve at present along that path.

2. THE HEPA-BETA LOOP
2.1. Physiology

The control of insulin secretion in normal man in the basal state is predominantly a function of the prevailing glucose concentration(7). This is not to deny that ketone bodies, amino-acids, hormones (eg. adrenaline, cortisol, glucagon) or gut or neural stimuli play a role, but simply to affirm that in the basal state glucose concentration is the major stimulus to continuing insulin secretion, while insulin is the major switching-hormone for glucose production and disposal(9). This can be represented as a dynamic interaction between the liver hepatocytes and the ß-cell, and has been termed the "hepa-beta" loop.

This feed-back loop is shown diagramatically in Figure 1. The predominant signal for insulin release is shown as the glucose concentration which has a positive effect on the ß-cell in the pancreas. Insulin and glucagon output are modulated by this signal and interact to control gluconeogenesis at the liver, and insulin also passes through the liver to control glucose clearance in the periphery.

Figure 1. Diagram of the "Hepa-beta" loop of insulin control of plasma glucose and the modulation of the pancreatic hormones by the prevailing glucose concentration.

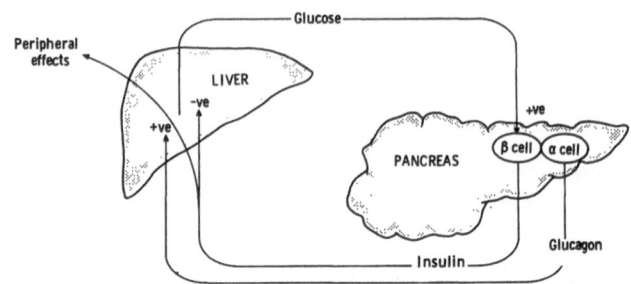

2.2. Practical Aspects

In juvenile onset diabetes one cannot optimise the feed-back loop as the ß-cells are defunct. However, in maturity-onset diabetics there are a variety of options open. The first is the possibility of augmentation of the ß-cell response by sulphonylurea therapy. If relatively more insulin is secreted for any given glycaemic stimulus then the blood glucose and other metabolites should move towards the normal homeostatic balance (10). Secondly, it is possible to augment the insulin concentrations directly by giving a long-acting insulin such as Ultralente which supplements the output of the ß-cell in the basal state (11). A third possibility is to increase the effectiveness of the insulin signal (ie. decrease insulin resistance). One consistently reliable way of achieving this is by weight reduction in overweight maturity-onset diabetics, and lowering blood glucose may have an effect in its own right (12).

3. PULSATILE INSULIN DELIVERY
3.1. Physiology

Insulin is produced in pulsations of 13-15 minutes in normal subjects (13). This may have implications in terms of differential

Figure 2. Plasma insulin profiles of a normal subject (upper panel) and diabetic subject (lower panel) with samples taken every minute, and data plotted as the mean +SEM of the three-minute moving average(14).

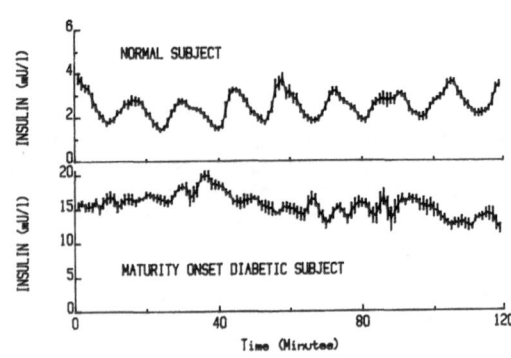

signalling to the liver and periphery, and may reflect some aspects of the fine control of insulin secretion. Interestingly, maturity onset diabetic subjects do not produce consistent oscillations of insulin secretion, even when the disease process is mild (ie. in those with near-normal fasting plasma glucose concentrations) (14). Two insulin secretory profiles are shown in Figure 2 - that of a normal subject (upper panel), which demonstrates regular secretory oscillations, and that of a non-insulin dependent diabetic subject (lower panel), showing a more chaotic, irregular profile:

The possibility remains that despite an adequate **quantity** of insulin secretion in maturity-onset diabetes, the **qualitative** aspects of its production are impaired and the loss of the pulsatile secretory pattern may interfere with its hypoglycaemic action. There is some evidence to support this, for in normal subjects, given somatostatin to suppresss their endogenous secretion, insulin given in an oscillatory fashion caused greater hypoglycaemia than that caused by an identical quantity of insulin infused steadily (Figure 3). Monocyte receptors were comparatively down-regulated in the case where steady insulin was given suggesting that constant exposure to insulin causes down-regulation (15).

Figure 3.
The contrasting effect of steady versus pulsatile insulin administration in a group of normal subjects given somatostatin and glucagon overnight. Lower panel: plasma glucose concentrations $\pm$ SEM. Upper panel: % insulin specifically bound to monocytes after overnight steady or pulsed insulin administration.

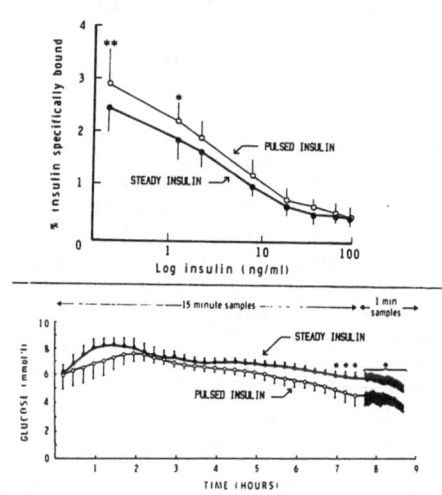

In addition, since insulin is a powerful hypoglycaemic agent, pulsations may allow time for a signal of given amplitude to act before further secretion. By analogy a Chef would always allow time for a spice to assimilate into a sauce and then would taste it before adding more. A similar quantal approach to insulin secretion might be a mechanism whereby the body prevents hypoglycaemia.

Insulin is cleared very rapidly from the plasma with a half-life of about 4 minutes (16). This is in very marked contrast to some other hormones, such as cortisol, which have much slower clearance rates. It is likely that the body has evolved such a fast removal simply because the hypoglycaemic effect of insulin is so powerful. One could then postulate on purely theoretical grounds that an optimal secretion time-interval would be about 3 half-lives or 12 minutes! Fig 4. shows the deconvolution of insulin concentrations into pancreatic insulin delivery and demonstrates the on-off nature of insulin secretion in man.

Figure 4. Upper panel: Plasma insulin concentration in a normal subject measured at 1 minute intervals for 150 minutes ± SEM of 3 minute moving average. Middle panel: Identical data to Upper panel but with logarithmic axis and with superimposed mono-exponential declinations assuming an insulin half life of 3.8 minutes. Lower panel: Resultant calculated insulin delivery rate which is a function of the spacing of the exponential declinations in the middle panel.

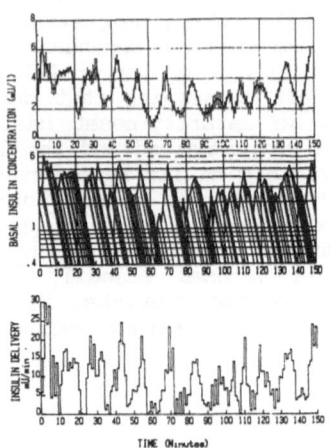

3.2. Practical Aspects

Pulsatile insulin delivery may have theoretical benefits in terms of relatively increased hypoglycaemic effect but in practice it is difficult to administer since it would need to be given intravenously (CIVII) using a cyclically switched pump. 15 minute pulsations given subcutaneously would be 'smoothed' by slow absorption so that the plasma concentrations would scarcely cycle at all. In addition, even if there were a 25% increase in hypoglycaemic effect of insulin when given in pulses in the basal state, this could be compensated for by an increase in steady insulin concentrations which could then be given more conveniently subcutaneously. At present we have no evidence that pulsations in the periphery are optimal, since one of the theoretical reasons for their evolution could be selective hepatic and peripheral signalling, whereby the liver responds to peaks and the periphery responds to mean concentrations (17). In practical terms one might adopt the pessimistic approach that physiological insulin oscillations cannot be reproduced in diabetic man. It is possible, however, that future generation implantable pumps may function better and require less insulin in a reservoir if glucose-sensing and insulin delivery is intermittant.

Nevertheless, the _ideal_ theoretical circumstances of insulin administration would be to give all of it as pure short-acting insulin which could be rapidly switched on or off to allow for sudden changes in exercise, temperature, meals or stress. In practice, however, the evidence shows that relying on short-acting insulin alone through CSII can lead to rapid and dangerous hyperglycaemia (18). Clearly it is necessary to temper enthusiasm for physiological exactness with due regard for the safety of patients (19). Perhaps pump therapy will be found to be safer when given against a background of long-acting insulin, such as Ultralente.

It is also possible that some patients with very high insulin requirements might benefit from intermittant administration. Those patients with established IV lines (in intensive care, for instance) may benefit from having insulin in pulses, since hepatic enlargement is a well described phenomenon in these patients if they are over-insulinised, and episodic insulin may allow one to reduce the total quantity of insulin given.

4. THE STIMULUS-EFFECTOR MIS-MATCH
4.1. Physiology

Insulin action and glucose disappearance are theoretically mis-matched. This is because insulin may take several minutes to have any detectable hypoglycaemic effect and this effect once started may continue long after plasma insulin concentrations have returned to normal. Glucose, on the other hand, may be rapidly absorbed and reach high plasma concentrations. If the high plasma concentration has a continuing effect on insulin secretion even while the glucose concentration is dropping then hypoglycaemia may occur. Both cephalic and first-phase responses help to circumvent the problem. Cephalic phase insulin, whereby insulin is secreted from vagal signals without any nutrient stimulus, allows for the time delay in cellular response to insulin (Fig 5). Hepatocytes and peripheral tissues may then be beginning to take up glucose when it first appears in the blood stream.

Figure 5. Plasma insulin profiles from a sheep. Upper panel: Fed at 45 minutes. Lower panel: Food shown but not consumed at 45 minutes. Data from 1 minute sampling ± SEM on the 3 minute moving average.

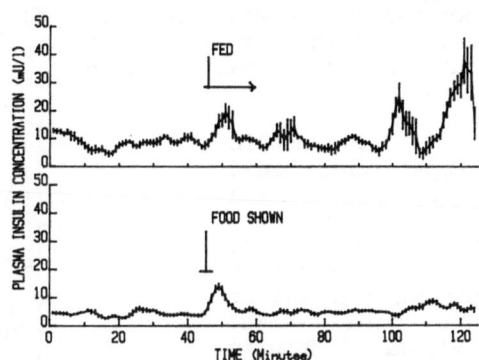

Similarly first-phase insulin allows a powerful insulin signal to be triggered on the basis of a sudden upward <u>change</u> of glucose concentration while second phase insulin is secreted more slowly in response to prevailing glucose <u>concentrations.</u>

4.2. Practical Aspects

Cephalic phase insulin secretion can be mimicked by subcutaneous insulin injections about 20 minutes before a meal. This allows time for insulin to be absorbed and acting before the nutrient load comes into the blood stream. If the injection is given after a meal the insulin appears to take much longer to act as it is then working on a background

136

of progressive hyperglycaemia. However, even optimally timed
subcutaneous injections of soluble insulin do not allow insulin
concentrations to rise as fast as they do in the normal population, and
insulin action therefore always tends to be delayed (20). It is this
delay that makes snacks between meals mandatory in juvenile onset
diabetes. One of the advantages of CSII insulin therapy is that rapid
adjustment of insulin concentrations can be made and thus allow for
erratic meal and exercise times. However, the time-course of first and
second-phase insulin secretion cannot be mimicked by any combination of
depot sub-cutaneous insulin and consequently one needs to advise
conventionally treated diabetics to avoid those situations where sudden
changes of insulin secretion might occur in normal subjects. In
practical terms this means avoidance of large glucose intake or rapidly
absorbable carbohydrate loads. This applies equally to juvenile-onset
diabetes (where insulin therapy will always be mismatched), and
maturity-onset diabetes (in whom first-phase responses are diminished or
absent). Dietary advice would then also be directed at using high fibre
diets to delay and smooth glucose absorption.

5. THE INSULIN PROFILE
5.1. Physiology
Attention has also been directed by some to the possibility that one
should normalise the insulin profile rather than concentrate entirely on
glycaemic excursions (21). The hope has also been, of course, that in
doing so normoglycaemia might be achieved. In analysing such a profile
it becomes apparent that about 50% of the insulin is "background" and
50% is secreted post-prandially (22). Figure 6 shows the marked
differences between the normal insulin profile and that of a diabetic
subject treated with twice daily insulin.

Figure 6. 24 hr insulin
profiles. Upper panel: Mean
plasma insulin concentration
of 8 normal subjects: the
dotted line shows the lowest
insulin concentration
achieved and encloses 44% of
the insulin area. Lower
panel: Plasma insulin
concentration in 6 diabetic
subjects treated with twice
daily soluble insulin. After
Holman and Turner (22) with
permission.

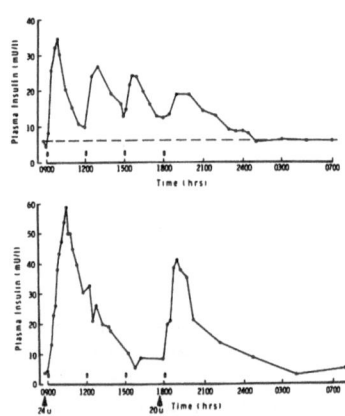

5.2. Practical aspects
A variety of regimens of insulin therapy have been proposed to
achieve this profile. They include soluble with isophane twice daily,
soluble with lente twice daily, lente twice daily with soluble three
times daily, and ultralente once daily with soluble twice or three times
daily. In addition, mixed insulins and preparations of intermediate

(and some would say indeterminate!) duration of action have been marketed. There are protagonists for all these regimens, but perhaps one can elucidate some general guidelines. First, in those patients who have residual insulin secretion (Type II and "honeymoon" Type I) it is sometimes possible to supplement background insulin alone and the obvious choice for this would be an ultralente insulin given once daily (23). In patients requiring full insulin therapy the background can also be given by ultralente and the meals 'covered' by soluble insulin - in this case 50% of the insulin would be ultralente and 50% split between the meals depending on their size. With insulins of intermediate duration (lente or isophane) the problem of the contribution to the basal levels is more complex since there is a fast-release component peaking 2-3 hrs post prandially when these insulins are used. Thus not all of the action of these insulins can be regarded as being basal and they therefore need to be given in a proportion greater than 50% so that there is not a run-out of insulin causing early morning hyperglycaemia. In practice, about 60 to 70% intermediate with 40 to 30% soluble may achieve this balance, and this contribution can be given twice daily again in a total amount dependent on the food intake and body build.

6. CAUTIONARY TALES

In diabetes it is never possible to manage all patients on one regime, however attached one is to it in principle. There are many confounding factors that make some insulins suitable for some patients and not for others. Mixing zinc insulin with soluble insulin may have quite marked effects on the absorption kinetics (24), blunting the short-acting component. Isophane insulin can be mixed with soluble insulin allowing some independence between short and long-acting components, but isophane insulin has the disadvantage of being too short acting to act reliably overnight (25), and insulin run-out is undoubtedly the commonest cause of the so-called 'dawn phenomenon' of morning hyperglycaemia (26). Some patients seem to manage on once-daily lente insulin while others have problems with run-out even on twice daily preparations, especially when given at 6pm with the next dose at 8am - thus hoping for a 14hr duration of action. Human insulins and their zinc derivatives seem to have a slightly shorter action than their porcine equivalents and warning of hypoglycaemia may therefore be less with human than with porcine and less with porcine than with bovine insulin. There is enormous day-to-day variation in the absorption of insulin even when injected into a similar site (27). Patients going into renal failure may have marked reduction in their insulin requirements (28), while infections or stress may double insulin needs for a while (29). Lastly one should always take the patient into account more than preconceptions of insulin physiology as is shown in Fig 7, where a 80hr profile was carried out on one patient to establish the cause of repeated hypoglycaemia. As can be seen, the hump of

138

insulin concentration (*) occurs at a point where no insulin was given
(by us!) and the patient then confessed, faced with the evidence, that
she had taken additional insulin herself. One should not underestimate
the psychological problems of the diabetic life-style (28).

Figure 7.
80hr profile on one diabetic
subject investigating the
cause of repeated hypo-
glycaemia. Top: Times of
meals given. Upper panel:
Insulin infused by pump.
Middle panel: Plasma insulin
concentrations measured.
Lower panel: Plasma glucose
concentrations measured.
H = symptomatic hypoglycaemia.
* in the middle panel shows
the time of an episode of
unexplained hyperinsulinaemia.
Bar shows time of
administration of continuous
low dose glucagon infusion.

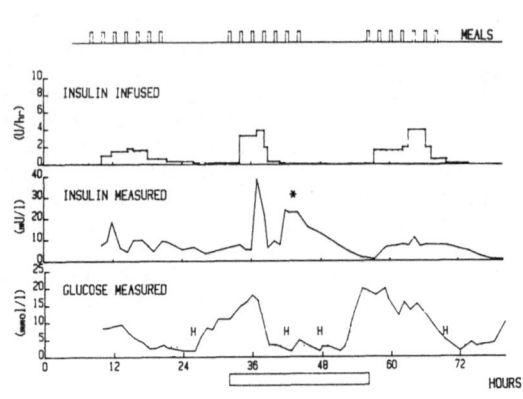

7. CONCLUSIONS

In conclusion, it is sensible to try to achieve near-normal
physiology in diabetes. But there are many individual idiosyncrasies of
insulin administration, absorption, clearance and action which cannot be
predicted from a general understanding of the physiology. Consequently
insulin administration regimes should start from physiological premises
and be based on the knowledge of how much insulin is required in the
normal state, and in what secretory pattern. The clinician should not,
however, be blind to the vagaries of individual patients, nor should
physiological principles be pursued at the cost of inconvenience or risk
to the patient. The aim of the physician should primarily be for
quality of life not quality of homeostatic physiology, though if the
latter can be achieved as well then it is possible we would see less of
the long term complications so prevalent in our clinics.

ACKNOWLEDGEMENTS
The help of Dr. R.C. Turner is gratefully acknowledged. This paper
was expertly prepared by Miss Rachel Church. DRM is Joan and Richard
Doll Fellow at Green College, Oxford.

REFERENCES

1. Pirat J. Diabète et complications dégénératives présentation d'une étude prospective portant sur 4400 cas observés entre 1947 et 1973.
Diabète et Metabolisme (Paris) 1977;3:97-107 and 245-256

2. Tchobroutsky G. Relation of diabetic control to development of microvascular complications.
Diabetologia 1978;15:143-152

3. Dornan TL, Mann JI, Turner RC. Factors protective against retinopathy in insulin-dependent diabetics free of retinopathy for 30 years.
British Medical Journal 1982;285:1073-1077

4. Barbosa J, Saner B. Do genetic factors play a role in the pathogenesis of diabetic microangiopathy?
Diabetologia 1984;27:487-492

5. Gorija Y, Bahoric A, Marliss EB, Zinman B, Albisser AM. The metabolic and hormonal responses to a mixed meal in unrestrained pancreatectomised dogs chronically treated by portal or peripheral insulin infusion.
Diabetologia 1981;21:58-64

6. Welborn TA, Wearne K. Coronary heart disease incidence and cardiovascular mortality in Busselton with reference to glucose and insulin concentrations.
Diabetes Care 1979;2:154-160

7. Turner RC, Matthews DR. Insulin Secretion in Type I and Type II diabetes.
Front Diabetes 4: 36-54 (Karger Basel 1984)

8. Horwitz DL, Starr JI, Mako ME, Blackard WG, Rubenstein AH. Proinsulin,insulin and c-peptide concentrations in human portal and peripheral blood.
J Clin Invest 1975;55:1278-1283.

9. Goodner CJ, Ham FG, Koerker DJ. Hepatic glucose production oscillates in synchrony with the islet secretory cycle in fasting rhesus monkeys.
Science 1982;215:1257-59.

10. Holman RR, Turner RC. Maintenance of basal plasma glucose and insulin concentrations in maturity-onset diabetes.
Diabetes 1979;28:227-230.

11. Turner RC, Phillips MA, Ward EA. Ultralente based insulin regimens
- clinical applications, advantages and disadvantages.
Acta Med Scand, Suppl 671:75-86 1983

12. Unger RH, Grundy S. Hyperglycaemia as an inducer as well as a
consequence of impaired islet cell function andinsulin resistance:
implications for the management of diabetes.
Diabetologia 1985;28:119-121

13. Matthews DR, Lang DA, Burnett M, Turner RC. Control of pulsatile
insulin secretion in man.
Diabetologia 1983;24:231-237.

14. Lang DA, Matthews DR, Burnett M, Turner RC. Brief,irregular
oscillations of basal plasma insulin and glucose concentrations in
diabetic man.
Diabetes 1981;30:435-439.

15. Matthews DR, Naylor BA, Jones RG, Ward GM, Turner RC. Pulsatile
insulin has greater hypoglycaemic effect than continuous delivery.
Diabetes. 1983;32:617-621.

16. Turner RC, Grayburn JA, Newman GB, Nabarro JDN. Measurement of the
insulin delivery rate in man.
J.Clin.Endocrinol.1971;33:279-286

17. Verdin E, Castillo M, Luyckx AS, Lefebvre PJ. Similar metabolic
effects of pulsatile versus continuous human delivery during
euglycaemic, hyperinsulinaemic glucose clamp in normal man.
Diabetes 1984;33:1169-1174

18. Ward JD. Continuous subcutaneous insulin infusion
(CSII):Therapeutic options.
Diabetic Medicine 1984;1:47-50

19. Acute mishaps during insulin pump treatment.
Lancet 1985;1:911-912

20. Nabarro JDN, Mustaffa BE, Morris DV, Walport MJ, Kurtz AB. Insulin
deficient diabetes.
Diabetologia 1979;16:5-12

21. Turner RC,Holman RR. Insulin rather than glucose homeostasis in the
pathology of diabetes.
Lancet 1976;41:1272-1274.

22. Holman RR, Turner RC. A practical guide to basal and prandial
insulin therapy.
Diabetic Medicine 1985;2:450-53

23. Phillips M, Simpson RW, Holman RR, Turner RC. A simple and rational twice daily insulin regime.
Quarterly Journal of Medicine 1979;191:493-506

24. Heine RJ, Bilo HJG, Sikkenk AC, Van der Veen EA. Mixing short and intermediate acting insulins in the syringe: effect on postprandial blood glucose concentrations in Type I diabetics.
British Medical Journal 1985;290:204-205

25. Ward GM et al. Comparison of two twice-daily insulin regimens: Soluble/Isophane and Ultralente/Soluble.
Diabetologia 1981;21:383-386

26. Gale EAM, Kurtz AB, Tattersall RB. In search of the Somogyi effect.
Lancet 1980;ii:279-282

27. Binder C, Lauritzen T, Pramming S, Deckert T. Pharmacokinetics of insulin.
Diabetes 1982 Ed E.N.Mngola. Excerpta Medica International Congress Series 600.

28. Tattersall RB. Diabetes, the young person, their family and the doctor.
Diabetes 1982 Ed E.N.Mngola. Excerpta Medica International Congress Series 600.

2.2.4. Diabetes Technology: From the pump to the microprocessor
A.M. Albisser and B.S. Leibel

INTRODUCTION

Eleven years ago the development of an artificial endocrine pancreas and its first experimental and clinical applications was described (1,2). An artificial pancreas is the dream of every insulin taking diabetic because it promises to replace the missing function of his pancreatic B-cells. In this regard, the device is capable of sensing blood glucose, of interpreting these signals, and of infusing appropriate amounts of insulin every minute of the day to accommodate all the metabolic requirements of feeding, fasting, stress and exercise (figure 1). The device presented in 1974 was the first demonstration that closed-loop control of blood glucose was feasible. The apparatus itself occupied a good portion of the patient's room itself, but elegantly demonstrated the feasibility of this approach which became known as the "closed-loop" system for controlling blood glucose (figure 2).

Numerous other groups throughout the world (in Australia, France, Japan, Germany and the United States) developed similar devices, one of which became a commercial success (Miles, Biostator) and was subsequently used in many laboratories for clinical studies involving the automatic control of blood glucose in diabetes. In 1974, all that seemed missing to realize this dream of the diabetic was to miniaturize each of the three major components including the glucose sensor, the computer and the insulin pump. Now a decade later, we are still awaiting a reliable miniaturized and implantable glucose sensor (3). Although we have available to us microminiature computer devices and miniaturized pumps, the reality of an implantable closed-loop system is not here yet.

The demonstration of this approach to managing diabetes stimulated many other groups to further develop pumping systems and the concept of the "open-loop" approach to treating diabetes was realized (figure 3). The "open-loop" system differs from the "closed-loop" system in that it does not incorporate within the loop a tissue, or blood glucose sensor or a computer. Open-loop systems involved infusions of insulin initially, intravenously, then subcutaneously and now even intraperitoneally. All these approaches are bringing closer to reality the opportunity of finer and perhaps better control of the disease. However, it is not known at the present time whether any of these approaches which succeed in lowering blood glucose and the clinical marker thereof, glycosylated hemoglobins, if implemented for long periods of time, will succeed in reducing the complications known to occur with the disease.

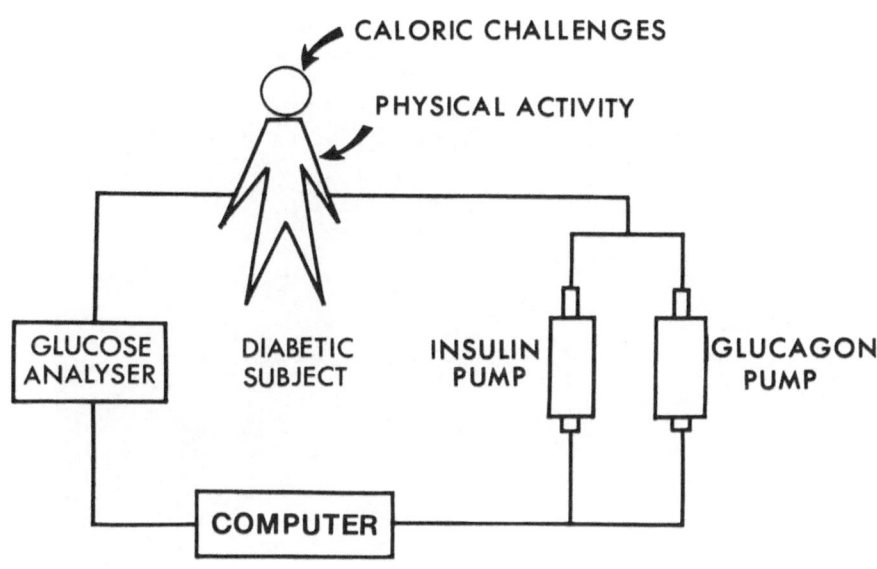

FIGURE 1. Closed loop insulin delivery system allows the diabetic subject unrestricted physical activity and dietary freedom because insulin (to lower blood glucose) or glucagon (to raise blood glucose) is infused under the direction of a computer which responds to signals from a blood glucose analyzer.

INTRAVENOUS INSULIN

In healthy individuals, the pancreas releases its insulin directly into the blood stream that goes into the liver. In this way, the pancreas can control liver function directly and assist in managing the disposition of absorbed food, which also follows this path. The major advantage of intravenous insulin delivery with pumps is that it approximates the healthy situation. However, access to the liver circulation is not as easy as access to the general circulation. For this reason, most intravenous insulin delivery systems developed to date and tried on human subjects have used the peripheral vasculature with catheters placed in the veins of the arm or neck, because they are easily accessible from the skin surface.

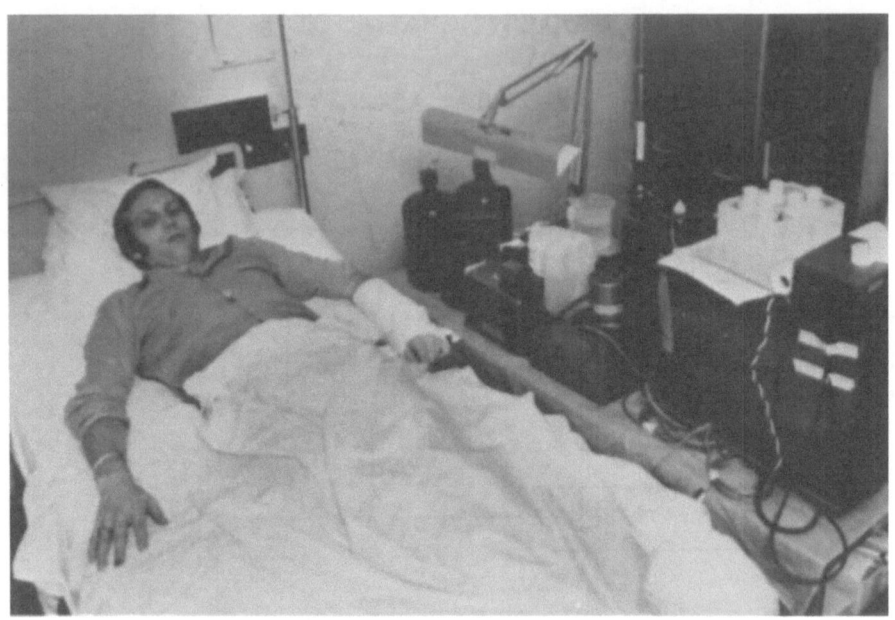

FIGURE 2. The first diabetic human volunteer to have his blood glucose controlled by an artificial pancreas.

Intravenous insulin has been shown to completely normalize the fasting blood glucose in Type I diabetics (2). By appropriate infusions at mealtime, intravenous insulin can also normalize the metabolic response to meals (4). Studies have shown that physical exercise before and after eating can be easily accommodated with intravenous insulin in such a way that both hypo- and hyperglycemia can be avoided (5). This advantage of intravenous insulin obtains because it does not form a depot of insulin that has to be absorbed gradually over time. The half-life of insulin in the circulation is about two minutes. It is much longer when injected subcutaneously or intraperitoneally.

SUBCUTANEOUS INSULIN

One of the main shortcomings of subcutaneous insulin injection is its gradual and perhaps unpredictable absorption. Because the studies with intravenous insulin showed that a steady background or basal insulin infusion was necessary to ensure normal fasting blood glucose levels in the morning, many groups attempted to simulate this require-

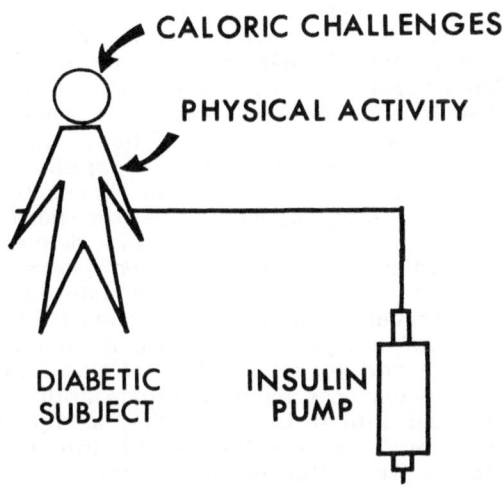

CALORIC CHALLENGES

PHYSICAL ACTIVITY

DIABETIC
SUBJECT

INSULIN
PUMP

FIGURE 3. Open loop insulin delivery provides the diabetic subject with a background or basal insulin infusion. To accommodate meals and snacks, additional insulin must be given by the patient via the insulin pump. Physical activity also necessitates changes in insulin.

ment by delivering insulin through a needle held in place under the skin in such a way that a constant background or basal rate could be provided, together with boluses at mealtime without additional needle injections. Although the first devices to accomplish this were rather cumbersome in nature (6), their application showed that a significant advantage could be obtained over one or two injections a day if patients were prepared to follow the requirements imposed by this mechanism for insulin delivery.

Pumps have now become smaller, some of them being approximately the size of a 1 cm thick business card. The improved control obtainable in this way approaches normal but carries with it the risk of developing hypoglycemia with exercise or at other times during the day or night. This risk is significantly increased especially if blood glucose levels are targeted to the normal levels that correspond with those seen in non-diabetic subjects. However, if these targets are relaxed to any great extent, then the resulting control is no better than that achievable by multiple daily injections of subcutaneous insulin (7).

INTRAPERITONEAL INSULIN

Because subcutaneous insulin injections or infusions are absorbed relatively slowly and because intravenous insulin presents a risk of catheter blockage due to the formation of blood clots, many investigators have elected to use the intraperitoneal route for insulin delivery (8). The peritoneum has a great capacity for absorbing insulin and other materials that appear therein. For example, people on peritoneal dialysis will absorb and exchange enormous amounts of fluid and other biochemicals through this route. Thus, the very small amounts of fluid infused by insulin pumps can be rapidly absorbed.

Many people believe that part of the insulin absorbed goes directly to the liver and in this way, approximates the normal situation even more closely than direct intravenous insulin delivery into the peripheral circulation. Studies by numerous investigators have shown that the rate of absorption of peritoneally administered insulin lies somewhere between the intravenous and subcutaneous routes.

One major advantage of the peritoneal route is that blood cannot gain access to the catheter and therefore clots of this nature will not form. However, the peritoneum does have an innate ability of isolating foreign materials introduced into it by producing a capsule that can cover the entire catheter and redirect the insulin infusion back outward from the peritoneum. When this occurs, diabetes control cannot be achieved and revisions have to be made either to remove and replace the catheter, or to excise the capsule that has formed. Further developments in the area of specialized catheters for this purpose may overcome these problems and the peritoneal route may become more popular for insulin delivery using either external or implantable devices.

OTHER ROUTES

There have been several studies in the last decade exploring other routes of insulin delivery. Perhaps the most interesting of these is the administration of insulin as a nasal spray. The first attempts to do this were relatively unsuccessful in that enormous amounts of insulin were required and very little was absorbed. In more recent studies insulin was mixed with a biological detergent and it was shown that somewhat larger amounts of insulin can be absorbed under these conditions (9). Some of the detergents cause a reaction on the mucous membranes of the nasal tract, but efforts to avoid these reactions may be successful and hopefully concurrently increase the efficiency of the absorption process.

Some investigators have endeavoured to encapsulate crystallized insulin in polymer capsules. Upon implantation, these capsules leach insulin at a slow rate and might in this way provide the background rate needed during the basal state when food absorption no longer progresses. One scientist has embedded magnetic particles in these capsules and has shown that by applying an external magnetic field, the release of insulin from these capsules can be accelerated (10). Since a pinch of insulin is literally enough to supply an adult's needs for a whole year, these implantable pellets, or injectable polymers of insulin are attractive, certainly in terms of their size.

THE PROBLEMS WITH INSULIN DELIVERY

As far as we can tell today, the major requirement in insulin replacement is to provide an exquisitively precise metering of the amounts of insulin needed. Clearly, too much insulin can result in very undesirable hypoglycemia and too little insulin inevitably produces hyperglycemia and in extreme circumstances, ketosis or even ketoacidosis. Our own work has shown that changes in the basal delivery rate of insulin by just ± 10% in the fasting condition is a sufficient change to result in serious hypoglycemia on the one hand and hyperglycemia beyond the renal threshold on the other.

All routes of insulin delivery have to deal with this metering requirement and where the absorption or delivery of insulin is unpredictable, one can be assured that the resulting blood glucose levels will also be unpredictable. The major problem in this entire area of endeavour is therefore how to produce a predictable and reliable way of delivering insulin. Many feel that a sensor is needed in order to eliminate the effects of this unpredictability.

SENSORS

Glucose sensors could in fact accurately control the rate of delivery of insulin increasing the rate when blood glucose begins to rise and decreasing the rate of delivery of insulin when the blood glucose level begins to fall. This type of mechanism which, of course, is the closed-loop system should get around the problems of unreliable insulin delivery or absorption. The problem with this concept is that glucose sensors are not yet available. Significant efforts to develop devices which will work either in the blood stream or in the subcutaneous tissue are progressing (3), but not as quickly as we would like. Should such a device become available, then this problem with insulin delivery might be solved and the entire device could be made small enough to be implanted.

INSULIN

For all these systems to work, it is essential that the insulin preparation used be totally stable during its period of storage in the device and during its passage through the pumping system and the delivery catheter. Unfortunately, to date, no entirely satisfactory insulin preparation exists for this purpose. Many of the insulin solutions when exposed to air or other materials, gradually deteriorate, forming large molecular weight aggregates that have reduced biological activity (11,12). Some of the insulin producing companies are working on this problem, but little if any, basic research is being done to address it directly. The main attempts so far, involve the addition of small amounts of detergent to the insulin preparations and the implementation of the concept that air must not be allowed to come in contact with insulin at any time. This of course, is rather difficult to do and we can only hope that answers to these problems will eventually be found.

CAPILLARY BLOOD GLUCOSE MONITORING

The two most significant advances in diabetes since the discovery of insulin in 1922 may well prove to be the introduction of intermediate-acting insulin preparations and the advent of capillary blood glucose self-monitoring. Today, it is the combination of these two major advances that provides the diabetic patient and his/her doctor with the tools for obtaining unprecedently good metabolic control. In the hands of a skilled practitioner, the valuable information made available from frequent daily capillary blood glucose monitoring can readily be exploited to optimize diabetes control not only with pumps but also with one or more injections of mixtures of short- and intermediate-acting insulin preparations.

Why then has diabetes control in practice only improved in the hands of some, while in the majority who monitor the blood glucose no significant improvement can be documented? This situation results because the valuable information produced by capillary blood glucose monitoring is in fact not fully exploited especially when the patient is confronted with deciding on his own doses. To remedy this situation, a remarkably simple approach to optimizing conventional insulin therapy in diabetes mellitus has recently been developed (14), using the modern techniques of artificial intelligence. This is a new technology based on control systems and information theory and which can only be implemented through the use of microprocessor and other computing devices. Thus, for those diabetics who are prepared to monitor their capillary blood glucose and inject insulin twice a day, but who are not willing to use a pump, a treatment scheme based on an insulin dosage computer now exists (figure 4).

INSULIN DOSAGE COMPUTER

Technology has assisted in bringing the sophisticated approaches realizable by artificially intelligent systems to bear on the problems of managing diabetes mellitus. Thus, it is now possible for a diabetic to feed information into a computer (see figure 5), which he can carry in his pocket. This elegant little device, because it has a large semi-conductor memory, is able to ascertain the patient's lifestyle and to optimize injection therapy based simply on four capillary blood glucose measurements per day. Preliminary clinical studies by Dr. A. Schiffrin in Montreal (14,15) and others have shown that diabetics using the device can remarkably improve their control within 3-6 weeks. Amelioration of control was achieved because mean blood glucose levels were reduced toward target levels, while concurrently metabolic variability was reduced. These changes were of course reflected by corresponding decreases in glycosylated hemoglobin levels. All this was accomplished without hypoglycemia or lifestyle changes and achieved simply by strategic adjustments in insulin injections taken just twice a day.

Although this new device does not meet the dream of the diabetic for an implantable device, it is an important practical step along the way, because for many patients it takes all the guess-work out of adjusting insulin doses. This "pocket doctor" promises to provide many insulin taking diabetics with a means for optimizing their on-going control on a day-to-day basis. Every effort in this direction is undeniably important, since good diabetic control remains the only alternative we have to avert the onset or delay the development of diabetic complications. In the meanwhile, research on many fronts continues in its quest for a cure.

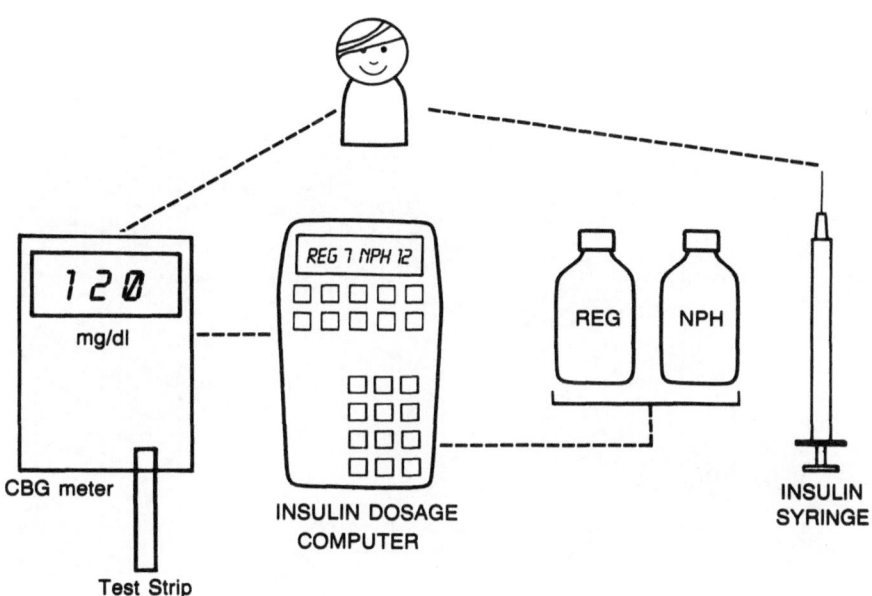

FIGURE 4. The insulin dosage computer brings to the patient for his/her personal use each and every day, the expert advice of the diabetologist. It takes the guess-work out of insulin dosage adjustments and restores good metabolic control.

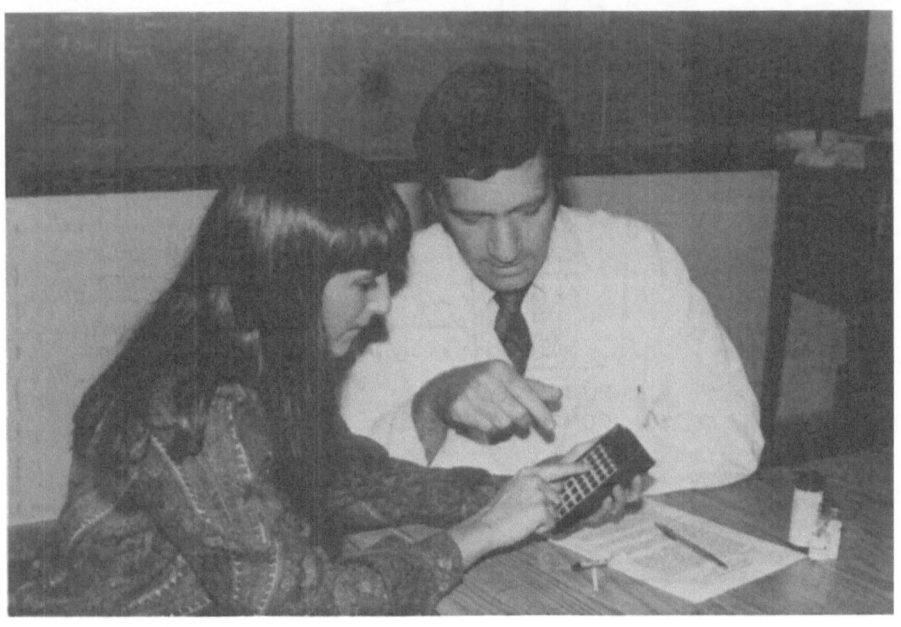

FIGURE 5. Using the insulin dosage computer is easy.

REFERENCES

1. Albisser AM, Leibel BS, Ewart TG, Davidovac Z, Botz CK, and Zingg W: An artificial endocrine pancreas. Diabetes 23: 389-396, 1974.
2. Albisser AM, Leibel BS, Ewart TG, Davidovac Z, Botz CK, Zingg W, Schipper H, and Gander R: Clinical control of diabetes by the artificial pancreas. Diabetes 23: 397-404, 1974.
3. Symposium on potentially implantable glucose sensors: Diabetes Care 5: 147-281, 1982.
4. Perlman K, Ehrlich RM, Filler RM, and Albisser AM: Waveform requirements for metabolic normalization with continuous intravenous insulin delivery in man. Diabetes 30: 710-717, 1981.
5. Nelson JD, Poussier P, Marliss EB, Albisser AM, Zinman B: The metabolic response of normal man and insulin infused diabetics to postprandial exercise. Am J Physiol 242: E309-E316, 1982.
6. Tamborlane WV, Sherwin RS, Genel M, Felig P: Reduction to normal of plasma glucose in juvenile diabetes by subcutaneous administration of insulin with a portable infusion pump. New Eng J Med 300: 573-578, 1979.
7. Schiffrin A, and Belmonte MM: Comparison between continuous subcutaneous insulin infusion and multiple injections of insulin. A one-year prospective study. Diabetes 31: 255-264, 1982.
8. Schade DS, and Eaton RP: The peritoneum: a potential insulin delivery route for a mechanical pancreas. Diabetes Care 3: 229-234, 1980.
9. Moses AC, Gordon GS, Carey MC, and Flier JS: Insulin administered intranasally as an insulin-bile salt aerosol: effectiveness and reproducibility in normal and diabetic subjects. Diabetes 32: 1040-1047, 1983.
10. Langer RS, Peppas NA: Present and future applications of biomaterials in controlled drug delivery systems. Biomaterials 2: 201-214, 1981.
11. Lougheed WD, Fischer U, Perlman K, and Albisser AM: A physiological solvent for crystalline insulin. Diabetologia 20: 51-53, 1981.
12. Lougheed WD, Albisser AM, Martindale HM, Chow JC, and Clement JR: Physical stability of insulin formulations. Diabetes 32: 424-432, 1983.
13. Symposium on home blood glucose monitoring. Diabetes Care 3: 57-186, 1980.
14. Schiffrin A, Albisser AM, Mihic M: Optimizing conventional insulin therapy using an insulin dosage computer (abstract). Diabetes 33 (Suppl. 1): 39A, 1984.
15. Schiffrin A, Mihic M, Leibel BS, and Albisser AM: Computer assisted insulin dosage adjustment. Diabetes Care, in press, 1985.

2.3. Pancreas transplantation

2.3.1. Introduction: Pancreas transplantation
H.H.P.J. Lemkes

INTRODUCTION
The first attempts to transplant pancreatic tissue in diabetic patients were reported at the end of the nineteenth century, so even before the discovery of insulin. Actually, these attempts represented trials in crude insulin replacement therapy, knowing about the at that time unidentified active principle in pancreatic tissue. These efforts failed because of lack of knowledge about vascular surgery and transplantation biology. They became irrelevant after the discovery of the insulin extraction procedure by Banting and Best.

Modern pancreas transplantation started about 20 years ago. During the following two decades transplantation surgery in general proved to be successful in various fields of medicine. It evoked high public interest and arose high expectations. Renal transplantation became a routine procedure in end-stage kidney disease. Heart and liver transplantation are nowadays accepted as life saving treatment modalities in selected cases of heart and liver disease.

Transplantation surgery has offered to the diabetologist the perspective of pancreas transplantation as a treatment which approaches a cure of diabetes. However, this concept was received with great scepticism. Much effort in diabetology has been directed towards the development of an artificial automatic pancreas. The potential use of such a "device" of natural sources was ignored. Unlike in renal, heart and liver transplantation, there was no urgent demand from physicians for organ transplantation in diabetes. Opposed to the sceptic silence in diabetology transplantation surgeons have exhibited a cautions and nowadays rapidly growing optimism.

SCEPTICISM
The first reason for scepticism referres to the nature of diabetes as a chronic disease. The impact of diabetes on the patient is two-fold. In daily life the patient has to live with dietary restrictions, insulin injections, awareness of the risks of hypoglycaemia. He experiences a restriction in his freedom of life style and may also experience periods of diminished physical well being due to metabolic derangements. At long term the diabetic patient may be faced with disabling complications of diabetes, like blindness, symptoms of periferal and autonomic neuropathy, cardiovascular or renal disease, lower leg amputations. Or he may not, since it is unpredictable which patients will reach these clinical end points of organ damage. These characteristics of diabetes as a chronic disease with an unpredictable outcome differ profoundly from the clinical situation in which renal, heart or liver transplantation are performed. The diabetic is not

facing a life threathening crisis. What is eventually to be gained from pancreas transplantation as compared with conventional methods of treatment, is an improvement in the quality of life, both in the burden placed on daily life and in the outlook of late complications. As a consequence, even the most excellent results of pancreas transplantation in terms of patient or graft survival are insufficient to justify such intervention. Ultimately, its motivation must be derived from sophisticated measurements of quality of life. Pancreas transplantation is still at the stage of improving technical results and so far, has hardly touched the problem of evaluation of qualitative effects.

A second reason for scepticism is given by numbers of patients and the availability of donor organs. One cannot imagine a future role of organ transplantation in the general treatment of a disease with a prevalence of about 2%. Most of the diabetic patients are to be excluded because of the non-insulin dependent nature of their diabetes. But even the insulin dependent minority outnumbers many times the most optimistic expectations on cadaveric donor organ availability or feasability of large scale living related organ donation. This mismatch of numbers disappointingly restricts the general concept of pancreas transplantation to a small selection of diabetic patients.

Thirdly, organ transplantation brings about the need for immunosuppressive therapy. The pancreas transplantation maintenance immunosuppression, including new drugs like ciclosporin, is not basically different from that in other transplantations. The obvious question is, whether it is justified to exchange the burden and risks of diabetes for those of long term immunosuppression. This question is unresolved. The same problem is encountered in immunosuppressive intervention trials at the onset of type I diabetes. Therefore, the most cautious attitude is to restrict pancreas transplantation to those diabetic patients, who have an indication for immunosuppression anyway i.c. to diabetic renal transplant patients.

However, if diabetic renal transplant patients are to be defined as the most important category of potential pancreas graft recipients, this implies a limitation to a group of diabetic patients with, generally speaking, advanced stages of diabetic complications. At that stage significant reversibility of organ damage is not to be expected. On the contrary, even some autonomic progression, independent of the succesful correction of diabetic metabolic state, is to be feared.

The only exception is found in the renal graft which is to be considered as a new start of an organ in the diabetic milieu. Recurrence of morphological manifestations of diabetic kidney disease is common in renal grafts and may even be accompagnied by clinical diabetic nephropathy. Protection of this new graft by pancreas transplantation seems worthwhile. But on the other hand, a second phase of end stage diabetic nephropathy is not to be expected before 10 or 20 years post-transplantation. Whether patient and pancreas graft survival rates will cover this period in a substantial proportion of the patients is doubtful at his moment.

OPTIMISM

The main reason for optimism is given by the technical results of pancreas transplantation during the past years. it is illustrated by the almost exponential rise in number of pancreas transplantations performed yearly all over the world. And also by the rapid increase in number of transplantation centres. After an early period of disappointing results, patient survival and one year graft survival are rapidly improving since 1980. Mean graft survival in the world transplantation registry for 1983 amounted 40%, but that included also the early poor results of numberous starting centres. In single experienced centres one year graft survival is over 50%. These results reflect a natural history in the development of a new transplantation procedure. The same curve was observed in early renal, heart and liver transplantation. It justifies the hope that within a few years the same successrate can be reached in pancreas transplantation as in these other forms of transplantation.

It also became clear that early poor patient survival was mainly due to patient selection criteria and not to the procedure itself. First transplantations were performed in almost terminally ill patients. The concept of pancreas transplantation is not based on life saving intervention. Thus, mortality in the first series mainly reflected the natural history in these patients. There is a trend towards earlier renal transplantation, and so synchronously towards earlier pancreas transplantation, in diabetic patients with end stage renal disease. Even living donor pancreas transplantation has entered the scope. Patient survival in these circumstances is excellent.

Graft survival rates are improving because of new approaches to the two main technical problems in pancreas transplantation: vascular thrombosis and exocrine function. Anticoagulation and anastomosis procedures are helpful to prevent thrombosis, although not completely. Ductobliteration or diversion of the exocrine secretion into bowel or bladder provide new solutions to the problem of exocrine secretion. Early detection of graft rejection, however, remains a major problem.

Graft survival is usually defined by insulin independency of the patient. Resumption of insulintherapy in a partially failing graft situation may be a subjective decision. So, graft function preferentially should be defined by persistent normoglycaemia. Statistical data with such stricter criterion is insufficient until now.

It becomes evident that pancreas transplantation as a safe and successful procedure is within reach. The next, most important question deserves now most attention: the effect on the quality of life of the patient. On this subject there are only casuistic reports. An improved physical well being, accellerated rehabilition, the wonderful experience of a life without daily diabetic troubles, all are reported enthousiastically but in a nonrandomised, uncontrolled fashion. This is even more important in the evaluation of the effect on the progression of diabetic organ damage in these patients. Casuistic observations are clearly insufficient to provide answers to this question. Long term randomised studies will be needed.

Progress in clinical pancreas transplantation has stimulated research in a field which is considered to be the natural extension or successor of organ transplantation: islet cell transplantation. The concept of islet cell transplantation is based on two major advantages. The surgical procedure will be almost trivial (a simple injection). Islet cell isolation will provide the opportunity of in vitro manipulation to lessen immunological barriers and to obtain larger amounts of transplantation material. The prospect is, undoubtly, fascinating. it would overcome all scepticism on pancreas transplantation. The present state, however, is still experimental.

LITERATURE

Sutherland DER, Kendall D, Goets FC and Najarian: Pancreas transplantation in man. In: The Diabetes Annual/1. pp. 198–216. Ed: KGMM Alberti, LP Krall; Elsevier Amsterdam 1985.

2.3.2. Current state of pancreas transplantation

P. McMaster, W.A. Jurewics, B.H. Gunson, R.M. Kirby

1. INTRODUCTION

It has been a matter of dispute for many years whether the credit for the discovery and development of Insulin should have rested with Banting and McCloud, or with their co-workers Best and Collett (1). Many Europeans, however, feel that the pioneering developments of the Rumanian Paulesco should have received wider recognition and perhaps if it has not been the misfortune of Paulesco to publish his work in French, the accolade of the discovery of Insulin might have been awarded to him. Banting and McCloud, however, culminated 20 years of intensive study, allowing the Ely Lilly company to manufacture "Isletin", later called Insulin, for the treatment of diabetes mellitus.

The spectacular impact of Insulin injections on children dying in diabetic coma received world-wide acclaim. For the first time, diabetes mellitus became a condition that clinicians felt they could treat effectively.

However, within a decade of the clinical introduction of Insulin, it became apparent that while the immediate manifestations of hyperglycaemia and ketoacidosis could be controlled, the disease was a far more complex disorder than had previously been recognised. We are at present still only in what must be considered the "second stage" in the treatment of diabetes mellitus which entails the extensive measures required to control the secondary complications of the disease (table 1).

TABLE 1. Secondary complications of diabetes.

Eye disorders
Renal failure
Vascular disorders
Sexual dysfunction
Autonomic nerve dysfunction

Six million diabetics are registered in the United States with an estimated total diabetic population approaching ten million. Approximately 3 000 deaths occur each year from renal diabetic glomerular sclerosis, respresenting 9% of all diabetic deaths, and nearly 48% of all deaths are in young insulin-requiring diabetics. Nearly one quarter of all dialysis programmes in the United States are occupied by diabetic patients (table 2).

TABLE 2. Proportion of renal failure diabetic patients

	Transplanted	Dialysis
Minnesota (1981)	38.3%	29.4%
Oklahoma V.A. (1982)		54 %
San Francisco V.A. (1982)		> 50 %

The position in other countries is often different. In the United Kingdom 600 000 diabetics are known, and there are around 12 000 deaths, and 500 patients entering renal failure each year. Of the 1491 new patients begun on dialysis treatment for endstage renal failure in the United Kingdom in 1981 only 5.5% of the intake were diabetic (2). This compares unfavourably with most other European countries.

The reason for these low acceptance rates are complex and while in some countries they reflect the overall low provision for endstage renal failure there is little doubt that uraemic diabetics often present a formidable clinical challenge.

Recent developments in dialysis, with the introduction of Continuous Ambulatory Peritoneal Dialysis have opened a new spectrum of treatment for diabetics in renal failure, although the outcome for conventional dialysis and transplantation remains disappointing. Transplantation between living related donors and recipients will give a 75% 2 year survival in experienced centres, comparing unfavourably with a 90% 2 year survival in non-diabetics (3).

Even in patients who are successfully transplanted there is a significantly excessive morbidity, attributable to their diabetes, which limits rehabilitation in nearly a quarter. Diabetics are particularly intolerant to steroids, and in one series, bone fractures were recorded in 69% of patients within 2 years of transplantation, major limb amputation in 31%, whilst 38% of patients went blind and 20% developed myocardial infarction (4).

Much of this high morbidity represents the late stage at which many patients are accepted for treatment. Braun (5) has recently emphasized again the very high risks that diabetics have, with over one-fifth of their patients having 70% occlusive coronary artery disease, and nearly 70% of these dying within one year.

The range of severe clinical problems in our own patients coming to transplantation is outlined in table 3.

TABLE 3. Diabetic patients

15 diabetics – diabetic 3-30 years

	%
Hypertension	93
Myocardial	80
Retinal	93
Peripheral Vascular	66
Neuropathic	50
Dialysis	100

2.   PANCREAS TRANSPLANTATION

It is therefore clear that there can be little ground for complacency in the treatment of the uraemic diabetic patient. It was in this group of patients that the first attempts at pancreas transplantation were undertaken by Kelly and Lillihei at the University of Minnesota in 1967 (6). Between 1966 and 1973 10 uraemic diabetic patients received pancreaticoduodenal grafts, 9 of which were undertaken simultaneously with a kidney graft. Four of these patients survived for more than one year but only one with a functioning graft.

The unsatisfactory outcome of this initial series convinced the University of Minnesota that combined grafting of the kidney and pancreas was inappropriate, and they therefore embarked upon a major series of diabetic kidney transplantation with subsequent pancreatic implantation. The major objectives outlined in this programme were:
1.   To resolve the clinical syndrome of diabetes mellitus and improve the quality of life.
2.   To improve carbohydrate control and delay or prevent microvascular complications.

The International Pancreas and Islet Transplant Registry to which all pancreatic transplants are reported, has shown a steady increase in activity since 1977. Although before that time only 60 patients underwent transplantation, over 500 patients have been grafted since then, 161 patients being transplanted during 1984 (figure 1).

2.1. Transplantation techniques

Great success at isolating and culturing islets from acinar pancreatic tissue has been achieved in the laboratory. In small animal models adequate numbers of islets can be harvested and successfully be re-implanted into diabetic strains, with the resolution of their disease. During the last decade a number of attempts have been made to transplant islets in man but out of 166 reported attempts that are known, only 7 patients remained insulin independent for 12 months and none are currently functioning (7). In addition there have been 3 deaths reported, 2 due to disseminated intravascular coagulopathy and one associated with hepatic failure (8). In spite of enormous laboratory promise, current techniques of Islet harvesting have led to a relatively low, impure yield of tissue which has not yet achieved successful endocrine replacement in man.

2.1.1.   Pancreatic organ transplantation

A variety of techniques have now been developed which allow the transfer of a segment or the whole of the pancreas from donor to recipient. These are capable of producing sufficient insulin to obviate the need for insulin injections. However, in all these developing techniques, the great weakness has remained with the exocrine secretion of the pancreatic graft, which in the uraemic and immunosuppressed patient runs a high risk of leakage and infection. The current techniques are outlined in table 4. In principle, anastamosis of the pancreatic duct to the intestine, stomach or bladder provides drainage

FIGURE 1.

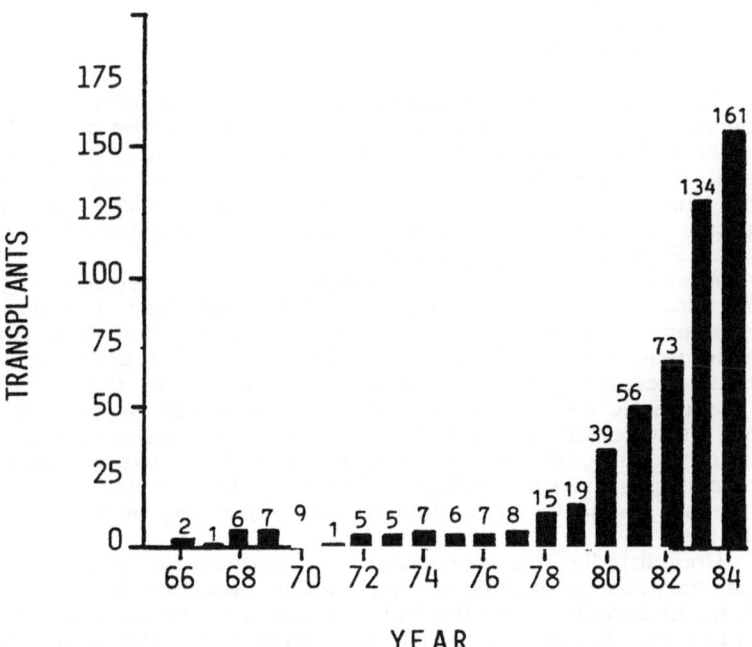

PANCREAS TRANSPLANTS

WEST.J.MED.1985

TABLE 4. Pancreas transplantation

Techniques

a. Duct drainage
1. Peritoneum
2. Intestinal/stomach
3. Bladder

b. Duct occlusion

with the prospect of long term satisfactory function. Nevertheless, in the majority of series, this has been associated with a significant breakdown and leakage rate with as many as 15% of grafts failing for technical reasons (table 5).

TABLE 5. Pancreas transplantation

Failures: Graft thrombosis
           Pancreatitis
           Preservation failure
           Sclerosis
           Fistula
           Rejection

The alternative approach of ductal occlusion developed by Dubernard et al. (9) offers a relatively simple technique using a latex polymer which produces flocculation and occlusion. Although the acinar tissue undergoes fibrosis, the islets themselves are spared in the early phase, but there is increasing evidence that this progressive sclerosis can lead to islet dysfunction in the long term (10).

2.1.2. Pancreatic graft failure

Whether whole pancreas transplantation or segmental grafting is undertaken, a haemodynamically unstable relatively low-flow situation is created. Studies by Calne et al. (11) show that flow through the splenic vein can be significantly increased if a distal arteriovenous fistula is created between the splenic artery and the splenic vein in the pancreatic tail. It was hoped that this would reduce the high incidence of vascular thrombosis which in one series accounted for 19.5% of failures (12). Other causes of graft failure have included pancreatitis and preservation failure (figure 2) but in the same series the commonest cause of graft failure was rejection, accounting for 41.5% of losses.

Undoubtedly the assessment and diagnosis of graft rejection continues to present problems. The sudden elevation in blood sugar in a patient undergoing simultaneous kidney and pancreatic grafting may in part be related to renal dysfunction or the administration of steroids. While a falling C-peptide serum level represents undoubted pancreatic graft failure the results are rarely available in time to be of clinical relevance. The newer techniques of angiography (13) and 111-Indium labelled platelet scanning (14) represent attempts to improve understanding and diagnosis of graft failure. In our series, by monitoring grafts with autologous Indium labelled platelets we found that primary graft trombosis represented the main problem, occurring more frequently than significant rejection in the first 2 - 3 postoperative weeks. The early detection of thrombus formation at an anastamosis site allowed the institution of appropriate therapy.

2.1.3. Carbohydrate control

Resolution of the clinical syndrome by pancreas transplantation can be impressive in patients who are established on normal diets without gross deviations in carbohydrate control for the first time. In the majority, carbohydrate profiles are normal and haemoglobin A1c levels are improved significantly. However, glucose tolerance tests and C-peptide responses show significant abnormalities, associated

FIGURE 2.

Graft Survival by Duct Management Technique

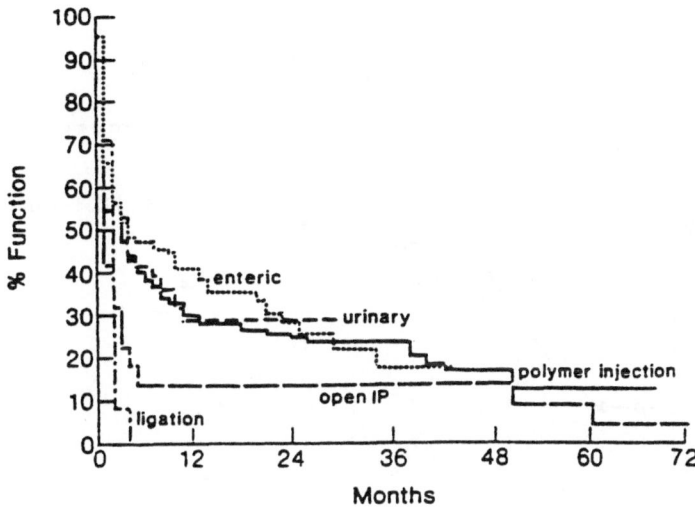

WEST.J.MED.1985

with a delay in absorption of glucose due to autonomic neuropathy, and a delayed response time by a pancreas which is both denervated and is draining systemically (figure 3). In addition, in the patient undergoing combined grafting modest impairment of renal function is still likely to be present, which further produces abnormalities in carbohydrate control, as shown by glucose tolerance tests. It is probably significant that in the Minnesota series where patients were transplanted before coming uraemic, detailed carbohydrate studies are essentially normal in the majority of patients.

3. RESULTS

The clinical results of pancreatic transplantation remain disappointing in spite of extensive effort and study in the last 15 years, but there has been a steady improvement in both patient and graft survival figures.

Of the 56 patients undergoing pancreatic transplantation between 1966 and 1977 only 40% survived for 12 months. Between 1972 and 1982 193 patients underwent transplantation and 72% were alive and well at one year. More recently, of the 276 patients grafted in 1983/1984, 77% were alive and well at the end of 12 months. This improvement in patient survival not only reflects increasing clinical sophistication in managing these difficult patients, but also the increasing acceptance of diabetics on to a transplant programme at an earlier stage in their disease. Improvement in graft survival has, however, been more modest (figure 4); only 40% of grafts are functioning at the end of 12 months using current techniques, and in some patients

FIGURE 3.

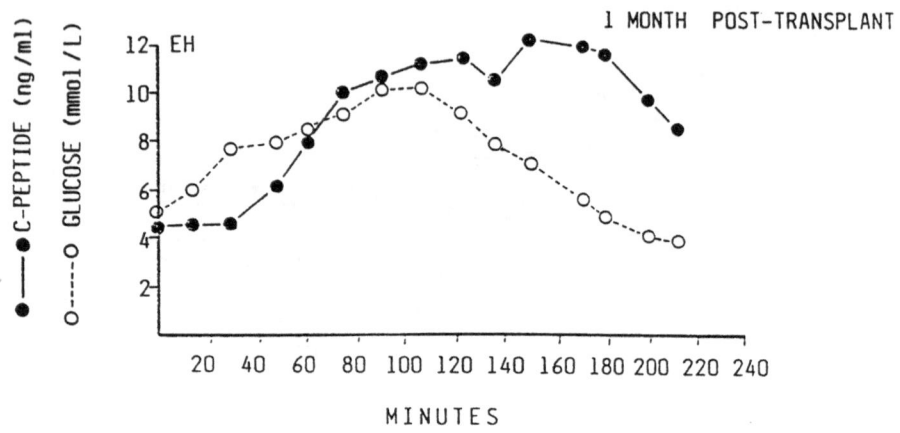

ORAL   GTTS   AND   C-PEPTIDE   RESPONSE

this is associated with significant morbidity. In our own uraemic patients undergoing combined kidney and pancreas transplantation,
wound infections with peritoneal leakage and peritonitis have been the
dominant post-operative problems leading to significant morbidity and
occurring in nearly one-third of patients. However, for the majority,
these were transient features which resolved promptly on appropriate
treatment.

In some institutions pancreas transplantation alone is performed
either prior to the development of endstage renal failure, or alternatively after a kidney has been well established and is functioning
without signs of rejection. The international registry data for patients between 1977 and 1984 state that following pancreas transplantation alone 26% of grafts can be expected to be functioning after one

year, and when the pancreas is transplanted following kidney grafting the one year graft survival is 28%. When the operations are carried out simultaneously, a perhaps somewhat surprising 35% will be functioning at one year.

A further major development in the last 5 years has been the introduction of Cyclosporin A, a non-steroid immunosuppressive agent, and there is increasing evidence that this is preferential in diabetics in whom steroids are badly tolerated. When the current results using Cyclosporin as the prime immunosuppressive agent were compared with historical Azathioprine controls, a significant improvement was found. Of 310 patients undergoing pancreas transplantation between 1977 and 1984, 39% had functioning grafts at one year compared with 182 patients undergoing transplantation with Azathioprine in whom only 21% had functioning grafts.

FIGURE 4.

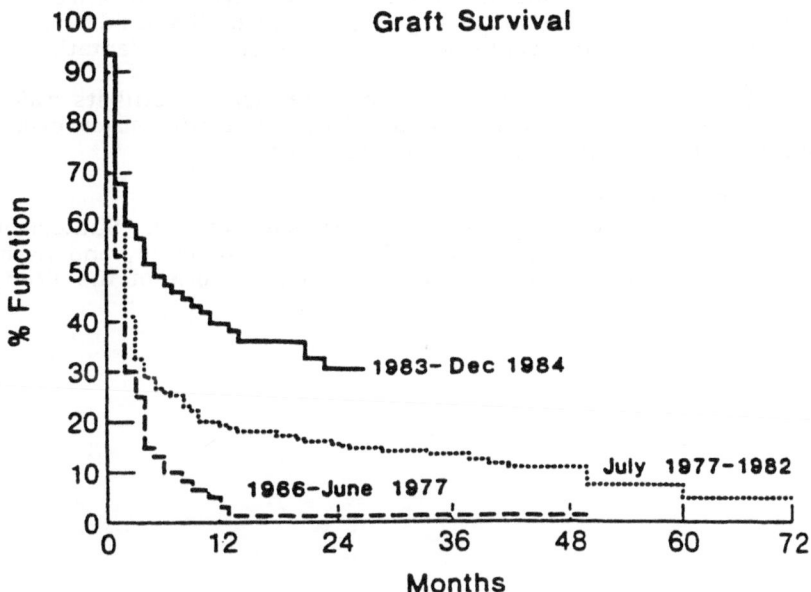

WEST. J. MED. 1985

If the overall results reported to the International Registry are disappointing, in several experienced centres nearly half of all pancreatic grafts will be functioning at one year. It seems likely, however that if further improvement is to be made, significant developments in technique must ensure that the relatively frequent technical failures are irradicated. Using a living-related donor rather than a cadaveric one appears to have marked advantages over cadaveric transplantation. Both donor and recipient can undergo a planned procedure at the optimal time and the recipient may be less likely to reject the pancreatic graft if they have previously accepted a kidney from the same donor. Survival rates of a technically successful graft from living related donors, have been improved, with 86% of recipients currently having functioning grafts. One interesting observation from Minnesota has been the development of isletitis in 3 out of 4 recipients of grafts from identical twin donors, reminiscent of the auto-immune induction of diabetes itself. In one of these patients the isletitis resolved with the administration of ALG treatment.

4. CONCLUSIONS

The development of clinical pancreas transplantation has been fraught both by the severity of the illness of the recipient, and major technical problems. In spite of this, improved results in both patient and graft survival have been achieved. At present the longest surviving patient with a functioning pancreas is over 7 years following grafting. Pancreas graft survival rates in diabetic endstage nephropathy patients and non-uraemic patients are very similar but the lower mortality in the non-endstage renal failure patients is encouraging, because it is of course in this group in whom the maximum benefit could theoretically be achieved if successful transplantation takes place.

It is clear that for pancreas transplantation to fulfil its main role of assisting the many thousands of diabetics with major problems, significant further improvements are required.

ACKNOWLEDGEMENTS

I gratefully acknowledge the permission of Dr. Sutherland to publish data from the International Transplant Registry, and permission of the Western Journal of Medicine to reproduce some of the Transplant Registry data figures.

REFERENCES
1. Bliss M: "The Discovery of Insulin" Edinburgh: pub. Paul Harris, 1983.
2. European Dialysis and Transplantation Association.
3. Sutherland DER, Fryd DS, Payne WD, Ascher N, Simmons RL, Najarian JS. (1985) Diabetic Nephropathy 4 (3), 123.
4. Surtherland DER, Bentley FR, Mauer SM, Menth L, Nylander W, Goetz FC, Barbosa J, Ascher N, Simmons RL, Najarian JS. (1984) Diabetic Nephropathy 3 (2), 39.
5. Braun NE, Phillips DF, Vidt DG, Novick AC, Nakamoto S, Popowmak KL, Paganini E, Magnusson M. (1984) Transplant. Proc. 17 (1), 307.
6. Kelly WD, Lillihei RC, Merkel FK, Idesuki Y and Goetz FC. (1967) Surgery 61, 827.
7. Sutherland DER, and Kendall D. (1985) Transplant. Proc. 17 (1), 307.
8. Mittal YK, Toledo-Pereyra LH, Parma M, Ramaswamy K, Puri UK, Cortez JA, Gordon D. (1981) Transplantation 31, 32.
9. Dubernard JM, Traeger J, Piatti ·PM, Gelet A, El Yafi S, Martin X, Devonec M, Henriet M, Karmel G, Canton F, Codas H and Touraine JL. (1985) Transplant. Proc. 17 (1), 312.
10. Gooszen HG, Bosman FT, van Schilfgaarde R (1984) Transplant. Proc. 16, 766.
11. Calne RY, McMaster P, Rolles K, Duffy TJ (1980) Transplant. Proc. 12 (4), 51.
12. Dubernard JM, Traeger J, Piatti PM, Gelet A, El Yafi S, Martin X, Devonec M, Hennet M, Kamel G, Canton F, Codas H, and Touraine JL. (1985) Transplant. Proc. 17 (1), 312.
13. Groth CG, Lundgren G, Amer P, Colleste H, Hardstedt C, Lewander R, Ostman J, Surg. Gynecol. Obstet. (1976), 143, 933.
14. Jurewicz WA, Buckels JAC, Dykes JGA, Chandler ST, Gunson BK, Hawker RJ, McCollum CN, McMaster P. (1985) Brit. J. Surg. 72, 228.

Index of subjects

A
Acromegaly 60,123
Activity
  physical - 85,86
Adrenocorticotropic hormone 67
Adrenal
  - gland 63,64
  - cortex 67
Adrenoreceptor
  alpha - 45,68
  beta - 45,68
Alcohol 83
Aminoacid
  - transport 124
  - uptake 125
Anastamosis of pancreatic
  duct 158
Artificial endocrine pancreas 142
Atherosclerosis 126
Autoimmune endocrine disorders
  2,5
Autoimmunity 11,13,14,20
Azathioprine 163

B
Biguanide 79,114
  phenformin 105,114,115
  metformin 107,114,115
  side effects 115
    gastrointestinal - 115
  primary failure 115
  secundary failure 115
Biological response 76
B lymfocyte 21
Body
  - weight 63
    - normalization 83
  - composition 63

C
Carbohydrate
  - production 50
  - utilization 50
  - control 160
Cardiovascular
  - disease 91
  - mortality 86,87
Cell mediated immunity 6,11,18
Cerebral disfunction 32
Chickenpox 12

Chromosome 18,19
Cirrhosis 125
Clamp
  euglycaemic - 80,111
Closed-loop system 142,147
Complement 18
Complications 4,107,121,131,142
  cardiovascular - 105
  diabetic - 103,112,152,153,156,
    157
  macrovascular - 85
  microvascular - 29,158
Congenital malformation 29
Corticosteroids 67
Corticotropin-releasing-factor 67
Counterregulatory hormones 60
  catecholamines 35,60
  cortisol 35,60
  glucagon 35,60
  growth hormone 35,60
  stress hormones 43
Coxsackie virus 4,5,12,13
Cushing's disease 36,60
Cyclosporin A 163
Cytomegalovirus 5,13

D
Dawn phenomenon 60,137
Diabetes
  clinic of - 2
  DIDMOAD 28
  experimental - 79
  heterogeneous - 1,11,27
  idiopathic - 28
  MODY 28
  type I/insulin dependent -
    1,11,20,28,33,36,51,60,83,86,
    124,132,144,153
    - a and b 20,22
  type II/non-insulin dependent -
    1,11,20,28,33,35,36,47,51,52,
    60,83,85,86,91,103,107,112,114,
    121,123,124,132,133
    compensated - 47
    decompensated - 50
Dialysis
  - treatment 157
Diet 77,83,86,91
  high carbohydrate - 91,93
  high fat - 91

high fiber – 93,136
hypocaloric – 91
low carbohydrate – 91
low fat – 91
prudent – 83
Dietary
- advice 84
- carbohydrate 84,91
lente – 84,93,95
- cereals 91
- fermentation 93
- fiber 77,84,91,93,95
viscous – 91,93
guar 91,92
- legumes 91,95,97
- preference 84
- protein 97
- P/S ratio 91
- regime 83
- rules 83
Digestion 93
DNA synthesis 124
Donor organ
cadaveric – 153,163
- from identical twins 164
living related – 153,163
Dose-response
- curve 80,110
- relationship 75
Down regulation 77,124,125,133

E
Encephalomyocarditis virus 4,13
Environmental factors 20
Epidemiology 12
Epinephrine 68
Exocrine pancreatic
- function 154
- secretion 158

F
Fasting 79
Fatty acid
- cycle 33,60
short chain volatile – 93
Feed back
- loop 50
- model 45,52
Feeding
- behavior 67
- control 63
Food intake 69,70
Foodstuffs for diabetics 84
Fructose 97

G
Gamma-interferon 19
Gastric emptying 41
Gastrointestinal
- motility 41
- peptides 41
Gene
immunoglobulin – 19
Kidd – 19
Lewis – 19
onco – 78
Genetic
- association 13
- contribution 18
- counselling 4,27
- marker 112
Glucagon 45,70
- release 67,68
- secretion 52
Glucagonoma 60
Glucocorticoid 77
- excess 123
Gluconeogenesis 75,114
Glucose
- absorption 114
blood – 67
- control 83,148
- normalization 83
- self-monitoring 147
- disappearance 135
- disposal 131
intravenous – tolerance test 39
oral – tolerance test 34,41
- oxidation 75
- potentiation 41,43,45,47,52
prestimulus – level 41,43,110, 131
- production 35,85,121,122,124, 125,131
- renal threshold 50
- responsiveness 43,47,110,111
- sensitivity 51,52
- sensor 142,147
- stimulation 39
- transport 79
- units 79
- uptake 35,75,76,114,115,124
Glycaemic
- index 84,95
- response 94
Glycogenesis 70,72,75,85
Glycogenolysis 68,72,75
Glycoside hydrolase

- inhibition 96
Graft
- failure 160
- function 154
hemodynamics of - 160
low-flow situation 160
arteriovenous fistula 160
pancreaticoduodenal - 158
- rejection 154,160
- thrombosis 154,160
Growth factors 78
Growth hormone 77
Gut hormones 35,43,45,67

H
HbA1c 121
Hepa-beta loop 131
Hepatocyte 124,125
HLA 3,4,30
- BW15 12
- DR3,4 7,13,18
- DR expression 19
Homeostatic mechanism 131
Hormone - receptor complex
- aggregation 77
- degradation 77
- internalization 77
Hyperglycaemia 50,52,131,147,
156,160
early morning - 137
Hyperinsulinaemia 77,123,124,
125,126
peripheral - 121
Hyperproinsulinaemia 123
Hypoglycaemia 18,87,113,114,
133,145,147
delayed - 58
spontaneous - 59
Hypoglycaemic
- action 112
- agents/drugs 83,86,103
oral - 77,83,85,87,104
other - 115,116
aspirin 115
ciglitazone 116
salicylates 115

Hypothalamic nuclei
dorsomedial - 69
lateral - 63,64,69
median eminence 63,67
paraventricular - 63,67,69
ventromedial - 63,64,69
Hypothalamus 63,69,70
- ventromedial lesion 123

I
Immune complexes 6
Immunological
- barrier 154
- etiology 5
Immunosuppression 13,30,153,163
Immunotherapy 8
Infectious mononucleosis 12
Influenza 12
Insulin
- absorption
variation in - 137,144
- action 1,35,75,79,109,111,114,
124,135
antilipolytic - 124
- antagonists 4
hormonal - 59
immunological - 58
metabolic - 60
- antibodies 35,58
- autoantibodies 17,58
- autoimmune syndrome 17
- binding 77,111
post - 77
bovine - 137
- clearance 133
- deficiency 1,131
- delivery
- by capsules 146
intranasally - 146
intraperitoneal - 146
peripheral - 134,143,144
portal - 122,134
pulsatile - 132,134
subcutaneous - 144
discovery of - 156
- dosage computer 148
- elimination 123
exogenous - 123
- gene 19
human - 137
intermediate-acting - 147
isophane - 137
long-acting - 132
mutant - 123
- output 47
porcine - 137
post-receptor
- defect 35
- loci 111
- preparation 147
- profile 136
- production 121
- pump 121
- receptor

- affinity 77
- α-subunit 77
- amino-acid sequence 78
- antibodies 18,34,58,59
- β-subunit 78
- biosynthesis 77
- insertion into membrane 77
- number 77
- occupancy 76
  spare - 76
- release 17,67,68
- replacement 147
- requirement 58
- reserve 4
- resistance 1,4,33,36,51,52, 58,77,78,121,123,124,125
  cellular - 75
  type A syndrome of - 78
- response 52,70
  early - 69
- responsiveness 75,76,77,111, 125
- secretion 1,34,36,39,43,47, 52,108,109,114,115,131,134
  phases of - 34,39,41,47,69, 135,136
  pulsatile - 34,122
  residual - 137
- sensitivity 33,35,52,75,76,77, 85,109,111,125
- synthesis 33
- therapy 2,86
- treatment 121
  zinc - 137
Insulinoma 123,124,125
Insulitis/isletitis 7,11,13,164
Interleukin-2 20
Islet cell antibody 3,4,6,11,16, 20,30
  complement fixing - 6,16
  cytotoxic - 17
  surface - 6,11,17
Islet of Langerhans
  A-cell 45
  B-cell 19,20,51,64
  cell mass 35
  D-cell 45
  hormones 63
  ions fluxes 109,110
Isoprenaline 107

K
Ketoacidosis 51,60,147,156

L
Lactic acidosis 87,105,114,115
Leprechaunism 123
Limbic system 63
Lipid
  blood - 97
  triglyceride 97
Lipogenesis 75,125
Lipolysis 75

M
Malabsorption 93
Meal
  - time 83
  - spacing 83
Measles 12
Mendelian inheritance 127
Mediator
  chemical - 76,79
Messenger
  second - 79
Metabolic
  - control 63,103,148,152
  - integrator 43,52
Metabolism
  carbohydrate - 45,93
  glucose - 111
  lipid - 93
Mice
  Balb/cBY 13
  Balb/cCUM 14
  DBA/2 13
Monoclonal antibodies 18,20
Mumps 5,12
Munchhausen syndrome 123
Muscle 125
Myotonic dystrophy 123

N
Near-normal physiology 138
Neonatal complications 29
Nervous system
  central - 63,69
  autonomic - 63,67,69,72
    parasympathetic - 63,64,67
      vagus 64
    sympathetic - 63,64,67,68
Nesidioblastosis 123
Neural
  - control 45
  - effects 41
  - factors 43
Neuro-endocrine
  - pathway 63

- system 63,67
Non-glucose stimuli 41,47,52,67
  arginine 42,67,110
Noradrenergic neurones 70
Norepinephrine 68,70
Normoglycaemia 121,131
  persistent - 154

O
Obesity 33,35,60,77,78,114,121,
  123,124,132
Occlusion
  pancreatic duct - 160
Open-loop system 142

P
Penetrance 27
Perinatal mortality 29
Peritonitis 162
pH 77
Pheochromocytoma 60
Phosphorylation 76,79
  de - 79
  - of serine 78
  - of thyrosine 78
Phosphotransferase 78
Preeclampsia 29
Pregnancy 28
Prostaglandin 45,115
Protein intake 98

Q
Quality of life 138,153,158

R
Rat
  - adipocytes 111
  diabetic - 69,78
Remission 4
Renal
  diabetic - disease
    recurrence of - 153
  - failure 30,156,157
  - function 98
Reovirus 4
Risk
  - factors 103
  - of type I 29,30
Rubella virus 5,12,13

S
Seasonal variation 3,12
Selection
  patient - 154
Serological studies 12

Serotonin 45
Signal translation 79
Spinal cord injury 123
Splanchnic nerve 69
Somogyi phenomenon 60
Somatostatin 45
Sucrose 83,84,97
Sulphonamide 103
Sulfonylurea(s) 79,103,104,107,108,
  132
  - drugs 51,52
    acetohexamide 112
    carbutamide 104
    chlorpropamide 88,104,107,110,
      112,113
    glibenclamide 87,88,107,112,
      113
    glyburide 111,112
    tolazamide 111,112
    tolbutamide 104,106,111
      - disposal 88
  extrapancreatic effects 110
  pancreatic effects 109
  primary failure 104
  secundary failure 116
  second generation 108
  side effects 112
    alcohol-induced flashing 112,
      113
    antidiuretic - 112
    gastrointestinal - 113
    skin rashes 113
Survival
  graft - 153,154,161
  patient - 153,154,161
Sweeteners
  artificial - 84
Synthalin 103

T
T-cell
  activated - 1820
  autoreactive - 19
  lymphocyte 13,14,18
  pancreatic B-cell specific -
    clones 20
  - subpopulations 6
Thyroid cell 19
Transplantation
  combined kidney and pancreas -
    162
  pancreas - 30,122,152,153,154
    156,158
    fetal - 69
    islet cell - 154,158

organ 158
renal – 153
Twins 7,11,164

U
UDGP study 85,86,104,105
UK prospective study 107

V
Vaccination 8
Vagal
  – response 41
  – pancreatic nerve 69
Vagus nerve 67
Varicella zoster virus 5
Viral
  – etiology 3
  – infections 4,13